Fourth Edition

WITHDRAWN

Winning the

Publications Game

The smart way to
write your paper
and get it published

Fourth Edition

Winning the Publications Game

The smart way to write your paper and get it published

Tim Albert

Author, Editor and Trainer, UK

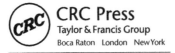

CRC Press
Taylor & Francis Group
Boca Raton   London   New York

CRC Press is an imprint of the
Taylor & Francis Group, an **informa** business

CRC Press
Taylor & Francis Group
6000 Broken Sound Parkway NW, Suite 300
Boca Raton, FL 33487-2742

© 2016 by Tim Albert
CRC Press is an imprint of Taylor & Francis Group, an Informa business

No claim to original U.S. Government works

Printed on acid-free paper
Version Date: 20151228

International Standard Book Number-13: 978-1-78523-011-0 (Paperback)

Visit the Taylor & Francis Web site at
http://www.taylorandfrancis.com

and the CRC Press Web site at
http://www.crcpress.com

Contents

Foreword to the fourth edition

It is six years since the last edition of this book appeared and about 30 years since editors started to obsess about the imminent death of medical journals as we know them. As things have turned out, the obituaries have been somewhat premature; the more things changed the more they have stayed the same. While electronic rather than paper-based processes have destabilised the publishing industry, what it takes for authors to progress from an idea to a citation has been refined but by no means revolutionised.

In consequence, Tim Albert's apparently light-hearted but in reality very serious analysis of how to get published is as pertinent now as when it first took shape in the context of a series of highly successful courses for authors. He shows that, regardless of technology, what still matters most is convincing an editor that your words are worthy of his or her journal's mission. His ten steps on how to succeed are two fewer than those of Alcoholics Anonymous but the chances of success are far greater. Half of those steps teach you how to know yourself: what are the self-imposed barriers to getting started? How do you translate complex ideas in your brain to straightforward words on a page? Why should academics and clinicians be unashamed of using techniques that are second nature in marketing and journalism? The other half provides ammunition on breaching editors' defences by demonstrating how to use the style and design of scientific papers that history shows they most appreciate – 'evidence-based writing'.

There is another way that this book is divided in two. Half the chapters are devoted to what authors need to do after they have collected their data but before writing a single word. Did you know, for example, that a successful paper has four key sentences, the first six words matter and there is likely to be just one of three conclusions? Or that a key to acceptance is to provide a single unambiguous identifiable message for readers? Or that a lengthy cycle ride along a towpath is the best way to mull over what to write (but only in the Netherlands)?

In the second set of steps, once you have the message defined, the target journal identified, the co-authors in agreement and the ethical committee placated, Tim Albert employs his long experience as editor, author and journalist to show you how to draft, redraft and obtain competent assistance from informal reviewers before hitting SEND on the submission system. During more than a decade as an editor I lost count of the times I wished an author had read *Winning the Publications Game* before sending me a paper that was confusing, incomprehensible, pointless or flatulent. The sole advantage was in wasting little time before hitting 'Reject'.

Harvey Marcovitch FRCP FRCPCH
Previously editor, reviewer and author
Now, reader
December 2015

Preface to the fourth edition

I find it hard to believe that it is two decades since I was first asked to help young doctors and scientists who wanted to write – and publish – a scientific paper. At the time I was a medical journalist with little formal scientific training who had just set up a small company running training courses on writing and other communication skills. I designed a course, started to deliver it, and found myself in an unfamiliar and unsettling world. What struck me was the large numbers of bright and enthusiastic people who came to my courses confused, depressed and often blocked from what should have been a fairly straightforward task.

This book is the result. The grand idea was not to overload the reader with lots of information and opinions from lots of different people, but to make things simple and straightforward. At its heart are 10 key steps, from understanding the (often unwritten) rules of the game, to sending off the completed article. The message I hope still rings clear: writing and getting published, despite what many people will want you to believe, is not a fiendishly difficult task. It requires a little organisation, a little thought, some simple techniques and a tiny bit of self-belief. *Winning the Publications Game* is unashamedly a motivational book, not a piece of scholarship, and I am reassured by how many people still tell me that it has helped them to write and publish.

My greatest difficulty in preparing this fourth edition has been trying to resist pressures to turn a short and helpful book into a long and unhelpful one. Since the book was first written, there has been an outpouring of research into what is now called 'journalology'. Most of it concerns what happens once an article has been written and there is little to help those who want to know how to approach the task of writing in the first place. And there has been one monumental change: the introduction of electronic publishing. We now read journals and study references on electronic devices, we write on screens, and when we submit we press a button and the content goes to our target journal. I have of course taken these processes into account, but in general I have been surprised how much the principles I first set out 20 years ago still hold true.

There are many people who helped me with the first three editions and their names are recorded in those books. I am still grateful to them. For this edition, however, I would like to single out Katrina Hulme-Cross from Radcliffe (now CRC Press) who commissioned it, and Harvey Marcovitch for writing the new Foreword. As ever, my wife Barbara supported me unfailingly as I disappeared yet again to work on this book. I would like to thank the 50-odd people in different parts of the world whom I have trained and licensed to teach my course who have also supported this venture and offered general advice and specific suggestions. Finally I would like to acknowledge my debt to the several thousand people who took part in what I estimate to have been 500 versions of the course, whose comments have sustained, amused, provoked and informed me over all these years. Their comments set the tone for each chapter.

Tim Albert
December 2015

About the author

Tim Albert trained as a journalist and worked for local, national and medical publications. In 1990 he retrained as a trainer, running courses for health professionals on writing and editing. His most popular course was on writing scientific articles, on which this book is based. He personally delivered the course about 500 times, which gave him plenty of information from which to develop and improve it. He has been a visiting fellow in medical writing at Southampton University, editorial training adviser to the *BMJ* and a council member of the Committee on Publication Ethics.

To the small band of colleagues (now friends) scattered throughout many parts of the world, who are teaching, under license, the course of the book.

1

Know the game

'Writing is really fun once you realise it is a big marketing game.'

The process of writing

The purpose of this book is to enable you to write, and then to have published, a scientific paper or article in a peer-reviewed journal – in other words to have your name on the established databases. It is not a book about how to 'do science', but a book on how to translate the science you do into publishable papers.

The driving force has come from what I have seen over more than two decades, while giving courses on effective writing to doctors and other scientists. What struck me was that:

1. many of them felt that they would be failures unless they became published authors
2. few of them had actually been given practical advice on how to become published authors.

Conspiracy theorists would have a field day. They would argue that those who have discovered the secret of publication are, for obvious reasons, unwilling to pass it onto younger rivals. That is clearly untrue. There is no shortage of senior scientists willing to devote much time to helping junior colleagues, and there are dozens of worthy books explaining in great detail the criteria for acceptable scientific articles.

Yet somehow all this energy achieves little, and many people who want to write remain confused and unable to start. To some extent this is a particular characteristic of science writing, which has become highly specialised and removed from other types of writing. Many 'experts' discuss in great detail exactly *what* conditions a 'good' article should fulfil; but few promote, or even seem aware of, some of the useful techniques for *how* to get started and write it.

However, there is a wealth of information on the *process* of writing, which is readily accessible to those who go outside the world of science into the world of professional communicators. That is the gap this book tries to fill, by treating writing tasks, quite simply, as writing tasks, and by applying the (mainstream) techniques and tricks of the professional writer to the (specialist) world of scientific writing. This may be considered radical, and some of the ideas may give offence. But I believe strongly that there are basic principles of effective writing that can be applied to all types of writing. It can work. As one participant once wrote to me: 'Before your course I'd had an article rejected by the *BMJ*. After the course I rewrote it and it was accepted by *The Lancet*.'

This book divides the process of writing into 10 easy steps. Some of the main problems that this book addresses, and the chapters where their resolution may be found, are given in Figure 1.1. What I hope shines through is that, despite the inevitable episodes of pain (such as these opening seven paragraphs which took more than 20 drafts), writing should be fun. It should also be rewarding and even liberating. This is not an impossible dream: it depends more than anything else on the writer's frame of mind, and therefore should be easy to fix.

If that sounds like one of those motivational books, so be it. That is precisely what I hope this book will be.

FIGURE 1.1 Common problems faced by writers

I don't have enough time to write	*see* Chapters 2, 3
I haven't got any good ideas	*see* Chapter 3
I don't know how to get started	*see* Chapter 3
I write too much	*see* Chapters 3, 4
I find it difficult to stop researching	*see* Chapter 4
I find it difficult to structure my writing	*see* Chapter 5
I find writing slow and painful	*see* Chapter 6
I make mistakes of spelling and/or grammar	*see* Chapter 7
I don't know when to write the title and abstract	*see* Chapter 8
Other people keep changing what I write	*see* Chapter 9
I don't know whom to send my article to	*see* Chapter 10
I don't know if I've written a good article	*see* Chapters 1, 10

The scientific article as truth

There are many different types of scientific writing (*see* Figure 1.2), but this book focuses on how to write an original scientific 'article', or 'paper' (the terms seem interchangeable). I have chosen to focus on them because they have become the main currency of scientific writing. They have also adopted a particular format, and on the face of it seem least likely to share common ground with other types of writing. In fact I believe the reverse is true: there are principles of effective writing that you

---

FIGURE 1.2 Different types of scientific writing

Original article	A new piece of knowledge we lay claim to (2000–3000 words, sometimes more)
Case report	A single event that could lead to a new piece of knowledge we could lay claim to (600 words)
Review article	Knowledge others have laid claim to (2000 words)
Systematic review	Organised analysis of knowledge that others have laid claim to (2000+ words)
Editorial	What I think of the knowledge that others have laid claim to (800 words)
Book review	What I think of a piece of knowledge that someone else is claiming (400 words)
Letter	What I think of the knowledge claims in your journal (400 words)
Distinguish from . . .	
Examination essay	What I can put down on paper, within a given time limit, about the various claims of knowledge from other people

can use to master scientific articles, and that you can also use for all other types of writing, including reports, letters, memos, grant submissions and patient information. This book will apply those principles.

Scientific articles have a long history. The first reviewed paper is generally considered to date from the middle of the 17th century, and a series of developments since (*see* Figure 1.3) has led to a process that is complex, sophisticated and international. The basic form of a scientific article consists of a 2000- to 3000-word report that normally addresses a single research question. It uses a standard structure of Introduction, Methods, Results and Discussion (the 'IMRAD' structure, of which more

---

FIGURE 1.3 Some key dates in the evolution of scientific publishing

1665	First scientific journals in France and the UK
1820s	First specialist journals
1870s	References began to be collected at the end of articles
1920s	First summaries appeared at the end of articles
1930s	First papers on the use of statistics
1950s	Widespread acceptance of the IMRAD format
1960s	Summaries at the end became abstracts at the beginning
1970s	Databases introduced
1980s	First international conference on peer review
1990s	Introduction of electronic journals and electronic submission
2000s	Growing concern about publication ethics, open access
2010s	Open access journals became established

later), plus other specific items, such as title, abstract and list of references. These articles are written in a particularly stylised form of English.

One or several authors submit an article to the editor of a journal. The editors have knowledge and integrity, according to the conventional view, and act as gatekeepers, selecting the 'good' and rejecting the 'bad'. They are assisted by a complex system of peer review, under which other people working in the same field are invited to give their opinion.

The criteria on which papers are accepted are generally considered to include the following:

- original: is the work new?
- significant: does it represent an important advance?
- first disclosure: has it appeared in print elsewhere?
- reproducible: can the work be repeated?
- ethical: has it met the agreed standards?

Each week thousands of these papers appear, in publications ranging from international general journals, sometimes run by multinational publishing groups, to small specialist journals published by a group of doctors in one country and who share a common professional interest. Most of these papers are now available on international databases, thus ensuring that, within a short period of completing the work, the findings are available throughout the world. Most of the journals are now publishing electronically.

The system is impressive. Week by week our knowledge grows as original articles – the basic building blocks of science – are approved, published and disseminated. It's a powerful thought and a comforting view.

The truth about scientific articles

It also happens to be a naive and unduly rosy view. Dr Stephen Lock, former editor of the *BMJ*, has written: 'The journals are serving the community poorly. Many articles are neither read nor cited; indeed many articles are poor. In general, medical journals seem to be of little practical help to clinicians facing problems at the bedside . . . Scientific articles have been hijacked away from their primary role of communicating scientific discovery to one of demonstrating academic activity. No more are grant-giving bodies basing awards on the quality of scientific research; the emphasis has switched to quantity.'[1]

The performance of journals does not always live up to the glowing picture painted of them. One major problem is that the peer-review system, for all its intricacies, does not guarantee that the bad will be weeded out or even that the good will be published in the most appropriate journal. There has been a small but steady stream of cases of authors copying data from a previously published article (plagiarism), publishing the same article twice (duplicate publication) or simply inventing data (fraud).

Nor do all the efforts of reviewing guarantee that papers will be good, as opposed to mediocre. The comments of others can be invaluable, but they can also have the effect of promoting conservatism and disparaging innovation. There is a danger that, by the time articles are passed for publication, they carry the stamp of agreement by committee and have lost any spark of originality. Most serious of all is the charge that the reviewers may provide unwitting bias on the one hand, and on the other downright chicanery (as one research team tries to discredit the results of a rival or use the information in a refereed paper to further its own research).

All this makes life extremely difficult as far as writers are concerned. Publication is not just a matter of adding to intellectual debate and seeing your name in print. Nowadays it is one of the main factors taken into account when assessing the worth – and funding – of individuals and research groups. This means that in recent years the pressure to publish is increasingly being replaced by pressure to publish in journals with high reputations.

Unfortunately, this can be extremely unfair, as illustrated by a story told by a young researcher on a course. She had written a paper which had been accepted for publication by a reputable journal. She scanned the journal for months – in vain. Eventually she telephoned the editorial staff. She was told that the article had been mislaid but, now that it had been found, it could not be published because the editor felt that the figures were now out of date. The author was heartbroken. In her eyes, she had fulfilled the criteria, but did not receive the kudos, or the points for her CV. At the same time the editor was well within his rights. If he felt that the readers would not be interested, it would have been wrong to have published it.

At heart is the harsh reality that our main method of validating science is ultimately based on a commercial system. Editors have many roles and have to reconcile many pressures (*see* Figure 1.4), but one of their main tasks is to ensure that the publication continues to exist. For this, articles must be read and cited. If this no longer happens, the journal will have to close. As Lawrence K Altman, a medical correspondent of *The New York Times*, has reminded us: 'Scientific journals represent scholarship. But they are also an industry. Medical and surgical journals in North America collect more than $3 billion in advertising revenue each year.'[2]

The traditional idea – that a 'good paper' will automatically receive the recognition it deserves – is clearly unrealistic. But where does this leave the aspiring writer?

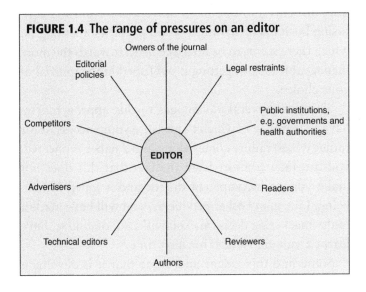

FIGURE 1.4 The range of pressures on an editor

Owners of the journal

Editorial policies

Legal restraints

Competitors

Public institutions, e.g. governments and health authorities

EDITOR

Advertisers

Readers

Technical editors

Reviewers

Authors

Marketing: a vulgar but comforting approach

The way out of this mess is to stop thinking of scientific papers as a means of assessing individual worth, and more as part of a commercial publishing system. Journals need good articles and every editor's ultimate nightmare is that there will not be enough copy to fill the journal. As a potential supplier, you have a marvellous opportunity: if you can provide the right product for the right market, you will achieve your sale – and be published.

This means redefining yourself as a supplier, your article as a product and your goal as convincing the customer (specifically: the editor) that he or she should 'buy' it. This allows you to move away from the confusing business of writing a 'good paper' (something on which there seems to be no agreement) towards the more manageable task of getting it published in the journal of your choice.

There are several advantages to this approach. You have a clear way in which to measure your success. If (or rather when) failure comes along and a paper is rejected, you can take comfort from the fact that this does not make you an incompetent doctor and a failed human being. Like many other producers, you will have made a faulty marketing decision. You will also, of course, have learnt a valuable lesson for next time.

Some find this vulgar and argue that it is devaluing science to talk about scientific papers in overtly commercial terms. It reflects reality. I am not encouraging you to write rubbish or to invent data; though I am encouraging you to see writing as a craft that can be learnt, not as a gift from the gods. Stripping away some of the mythology surrounding scientific papers and the world of journals should encourage more and more writers to have a go. And this in turn should raise standards.

Implications for the reader of this book

What this means for you, as an intending writer, is that you should stop being intimidated by those who appear to be more successful at writing than you. Take them less seriously; treat the writing business as a game. The rules are simple: when you have written a paper that has been published in your journal of first choice, you are the winner.

 CHECKPOINT

Before proceeding to Chapter 2 you should understand that you can win the publications game by becoming a published author. Do not let others discourage you.

BOOKCHOICE: An editor's view of the game

Smith R (2006) *The Trouble with Medical Journals.* Royal Society of Medicine Press, London.

In the first two editions I recommended a book published in 1991 and edited by Stephen Lock, outgoing editor of the *BMJ*.[1] In the review I quoted the contribution by Richard Smith, the incoming editor. 'I believe that the future for general medical journals – particularly those published in English – is bright,' he wrote. 'They will undoubtedly change but they will not disappear. Electronic forms of publishing will become increasingly important after a hesitant start, but general journals will continue to exist in hardcopy ... Indeed, the buffeting and transforming of the medical profession over the next few decades will return general medical journals to their central function of gluing the profession together.'

A decade and a half of being editor seems to have blighted his optimism. In a second book, published after he had left the *BMJ*, Smith concludes that 'medical journals have many problems and need reform'. Among these problems is the precariousness of the peer-review system: 'a flawed process full of easily identifiable defences with little evidence that it works'. He also discusses the dangerous influence of the various self-interested groups involved, such as editors (who want to increase their journal's impact factor), pharmaceutical companies (who want to increase sales) and authors (who need to get their articles published in prestigious places). This has led to all kinds of unethical practices, like people writing the same article twice, or pretending to be authors when they are not, or just making up the data they think would be nice to see.[3–5]

How will reading Smith's book help the beginning writer? Well, it should at least give a more realistic perspective. As he writes, '. . . scientists may have been victims of their own rhetoric: they have fooled themselves that science is a wholly objective enterprise unsullied by the usual human subjectivity and imperfections. It isn't. It is a human activity.' These words will be worth bearing in mind as you go through the often painful publication process.

2

Know yourself

'I think I'd rather go fishing.'

Do you really want to write?

The most important component of a scientific paper is not the data. It is you.

If you seriously wish to become a published author, you will have to make certain changes in your life. You will face added hours of solitary work and many frustrations. You will have to call on reserves of tact, optimism and determination. At one stage you could even discover that you are creating a monster that is threatening to take over parts of your life (and the lives of your loved ones).

Not surprisingly, many people drop out along the way. They end up with half-finished manuscripts, or a head-full of promising ideas that go around and around – but never forward. They may well be those who are loudest in telling you exactly how you should be writing. They may appear contemptuous of anything anyone else has written, but in reality this serves to disguise the fact that they wish that they had got there first.

What marks out a writer from the rest of the world is simple: the writer has found time to start – and finish – the writing task. The key factor is not so much knowledge or skills but time management. Successful authors are those who have managed their resources more effectively.

As a starting point, you must be absolutely clear why you want to be published in the first place. This is one of those deceptively simple questions that, once you have dared to pose it, brings out all kinds of motives that might have been better unroused.

The most common motive is one that people tend to be embarrassed about: publication is necessary to advance your career. There is no need to be ashamed. This is a fact of contemporary life, and if you don't compete you will lose out. Whether you approve of it or not is irrelevant.

Some writers say that their motive is to share with others what they have discovered. Others take a self-exploratory view: writing a paper is a test of self-worth. Or, as with climbing mountains, they do it simply because the challenge is there. There are the missionaries, who take the position that they have a duty to write because everyone else is publishing rubbish. And there are those who realise that they owe it to their 'subjects'.

Whichever motives you choose to admit to in public, in private you must be completely honest with yourself. Unless you know why you want to publish, how can you gauge whether you are progressing towards your goals?

I fondly remember one course participant who said after the second day that he had greatly enjoyed himself and learnt a great deal about the mechanics of writing a paper. But, he continued, he had a busy and successful practice and a growing family, and he had now come to the conclusion that he would make a better use of his time by going fishing instead.

He was in control.

Goals – and can you achieve them?

Once you know why you feel you should be writing, you can start setting some realistic writing goals. If you want to be a professor before the age of 35, for instance, you may decide that you need to have published three papers in prestigious journals within the next year. If you wish to write one paper for your CV then a different set of actions would be in order (*see* Figure 2.1).

Make sure that you are in a position to do what you need to do. You have a problem, for instance, if you need to publish an original paper and the material you have is only suitable for a case report. You may have to set up your own research, or find a new job where you can spend more time on research. But modern life is not always as straightforward as that, and you may not be able to take such drastic action. Furthermore, you may be part of a larger team and have little influence on what you can write. The important thing is that you keep a sense of reality: do not write yourself off as an incompetent writer when in fact, through no fault of your own, you have nothing suitable to write about.

FIGURE 2.1 Setting your writing goal

Version A: What is your writing goal?

Three papers in prestigious journals within the next 12 months so that I can become a professor before the age of 35.

What can you provide?

Study A provisionally accepted; study B just finishing final draft; study C needs final data.

How will you find time to write?

Fifteen minutes every evening before going to bed, and 2 hours on Sunday morning.

What are your writing objectives for the next 6 months?

1. Amend article A, provisionally accepted by *The Lancet*, and send off within 1 week
2. Write letter to editor for article B.
3. Send article B, plus letter to editor, to co-authors for final approval within 2 weeks.
4. Set the brief on article C within 4 weeks.
5. Review within 6 weeks.

Version B: What is your writing goal?

Bolster my CV with one article in a reasonable journal.

What can you provide?

One case history. Possible major study with two other centres.

How will you find time to write?

Two weeks between jobs. Then one evening a week.

What are your writing objectives for the next 6 months?

1. Decide whether to do the case history or the major study.
2. Make appointment with head of department to seek advice.
3. Buy new laptop.
4. Finish this book.
5. Review in 3 months.

Making time

How are you going to find time? Writing will always use more of this scarce commodity than you expect. We all share the set quota of 24 hours a day; what distinguishes us from each other is how we decide to fill these hours. This will inevitably mean that something must go.

You may find it less painful if you can keep writing tasks to a set time each week. This will help you to get into a routine. Many successful writers manage to do without some of their sleep, and get up, say, at five in the morning. You might find this too drastic, but you could go without a favourite television programme or put aside a couple of hours a week on a Sunday evening. Don't feel you have to allocate huge chunks of time. Fifteen minutes a day, 6 days a week will help you to make steady progress; it should also help you to maintain your enthusiasm.

Some people say they will find time when they need to. This is not a recommended option, mainly because there is an easier way.

Setting objectives

Now that you know what you need to write, and how you will find the necessary time, all that remains is to spend a little time deciding what you have to do to get there. These twin tasks will be your objectives.

Do not confuse objectives with vague ambitions. Most people, when asked to suggest their writing objectives, come up with enormous tasks such as:

- write three papers within 6 months
- finish my PhD before the holidays
- get something (anything!) published within 2 years.

Make your objectives attainable. They could be simple tasks, like reading the *Instructions to authors* from a target journal, or reading a book (or perhaps just finishing this one), or drawing up some tables from your data. These are all tasks that you will need to complete, and you will find life much more satisfying if you make steady progress – and can acknowledge that fact.

Put a realistic time limit on each objective, and a time limit, such as 6 months or a year, on the whole series. Make time to review these regularly. After a few months you will start to realise that you are beginning to achieve what you set out to achieve. After a year you could well be surprised by how far you have come.

---

❷ CHECKPOINT

Before proceeding to Chapter 3 you should be absolutely clear why you want to write, how you can achieve this goal and when you will achieve it. Write it down.

3

First set yourself a brief

'The key point is the need for a message – and this can take as long as 2–3 hours to finalise, even when you know all the results.'

When to stop researching and start writing

One of the main reasons why writing fails is that the reader cannot find a clear message. This is usually because the writer has failed to put one in, probably because he or she started to write too early. Good writing is rooted in good thought, and this preparatory stage, which involves taking time to think about what you are writing, is vital. It is often neglected.

If you have got this far you presumably have some idea of what you wish to write. You may only have a hypothesis or a protocol; on the other hand your kitchen table may well be groaning with data. Resist the temptation to go straight to the word processor and do not believe those who say you should start putting your ideas on paper as soon as possible. 'Do a literature search and try sketching in some of the Introduction,' they might say, or 'Write down what you have done so far for the Methods. Perhaps you can jot down some ideas on the harder bits, like the Discussion, and before you know where you are, you've nearly finished . . .'

This is not a sensible way to proceed. With no clear vision, you will become obsessed with detail. You will fiddle with figures, chase up obscure references and have long disputes with your colleagues over everything from statistics to style. At best this will delay and demoralise; at worst it will destroy the whole project.

You wouldn't dream of behaving in this way when you drive a car. You don't jump in and start driving. You work out where your destination is and the best route for getting there. All sensible business people do comprehensive planning and market research before launching a new product, yet all over the world doctors and researchers invest time and egos in writing papers that – were they to think them through properly from the start – they would realise still have major flaws.

Set aside some time to think and make this a formal part of the process. I call this stage 'setting the brief' (a term that comes from the jargon of journalism). Some people do this informally, or even subconsciously, but I recommend that it becomes a major ritual, to be undertaken at the start of any substantial writing project. Take as much time as you need – and make sure that you commit your decisions to paper. Once you have completed it, you will be through the worst and you will have made decisions in five key areas:

1. the message
2. the market
3. the length
4. the deadline
5. the co-authors.

This process of setting the brief marks the time when the research ends and the writing starts. You will, of course, revisit your data, but the relationship between research and writing has subtly changed. From now on the piece of writing becomes the master, and the data its servant.

FIGURE 3.1 Caution to writers

Do *not* start defining the brief unless you can answer yes to the following questions.

- Is the data collection at a stage which allows me to make generalisations?
- Have I obtained approval from the appropriate ethical committee, or a letter from an appropriate body saying it is not required?
- Has the study (if a randomised controlled trial) been registered as a clinical trial?
- Have I obtained the appropriate guidelines (such as CONSORT for randomised controlled trials or STROBE for observational studies)? (For further information on these guidelines: www.equator-network.org)
- Do I have the consent of the other researchers to start writing this up?

This is the best way of ensuring that, at the end of the process, you will have written something that is clear, consistent and coherent.

Finally, a word of caution: there are some basic conditions that you must meet if the article is to get published (*see* Figure 3.1). If you cannot answer yes to each question, you should pause awhile – and try to meet them. If you can't – for example, the statistician tells you that your sample size cannot justify any conclusions, or the ethics committee says you cannot do this work – you should seriously consider aborting the project, and working on something that is going to be (more) achievable.

Only one message per article

Scientific papers are expected to communicate findings to other people. To do this successfully, you need to do more than throw a number of facts onto a piece of paper. You need to organise or structure them, so that the relationship between the various items of information becomes clear. If you organise successfully, there will be a common theme, which the reader will be able to pull out as a single thought. This is your message.

The problem with any piece of research, and any piece of writing, is that the number of potential messages is vast. Many people try to skirt round the challenge of working out which is the most important, or they try to fit them all in anyway. That is why so much writing fails and the reader is unable to come away with a clear message. Readers usually blame themselves for not being clever enough to understand, but almost always the fault lies with the writer.

Do not expect a clear message to emerge as you write (unless you are a medical sociologist, because you have probably been taught the opposite). This is like putting a pile of bricks together and expecting a house to arise. There is only one way of ensuring that your writing is focused on one simple message and that is by defining this message carefully before you start. To keep it as clear as possible, you should express it as a simple sentence of 10–14 words, with a verb.

Imagine, for example, that you have spent the past 5 years conducting a trial to see whether Obecalp is an effective treatment for post-lunchtime amnesia in doctors. You may think the results are so momentous that you couldn't possibly confine them to one sentence. But try, and you will immediately, and with little difficulty, come up with a number of alternatives.

1. Obecalp is an effective treatment for post-lunchtime amnesia.
2. Obecalp is an effective treatment for post-lunchtime amnesia in doctors if given within 48 hours of onset.
3. This latest piece of research adds to the evidence that Obecalp may be an effective treatment.
4. Obecalp doesn't have any advantage over existing treatment (or, if you are not in thrall to a pharmaceutical company: Obecalp doesn't work).

All could be perfectly good messages for a piece of writing. All are plausible and, presumably, supported by the evidence. The information will, broadly speaking, be the same for each. But the exact form your writing takes will vary tremendously, depending on which message you choose to convey.

Making this decision is not an easy task. It should not be done in a darkened room facing a word processor or blank piece of paper. It should be done in what Henriette Anne Klauser calls 'rumination time',[6] on the move – travelling to work, riding a bicycle or sitting in the bath. It needs a clear(ish) head, a moderate amount of time, a pencil and a scrap of paper (used envelopes are particularly suitable) on which you will write down your thoughts. Feel free to talk your ideas through with other people – but remember that you are the one who is going to do the writing, and you are the one who has to decide on the message. (*See also* Bookchoice, p. 69.)

Use the language of the public house or coffee house rather than the academic journal. Far from limiting thought, this should clarify it. Which version is more specific: 'Obecalp is now clearly indicated as the treatment of choice for post-lunchtime amnesia', or one of the following?

1. Doctors should immediately prescribe Obecalp to all those suffering from post-lunchtime amnesia.
2. Researchers need to test Obecalp on more people before we can decide whether we should use it.
3. Obecalp cured three of the four rats with post-lunchtime amnesia.
4. Obecalp is rubbish.

FIGURE 3.2 Titles versus messages

On the left are titles published in the *BMJ* (5 August 2006). At that time the *BMJ* published short news items about these papers at the front of the journal, and these are shown on the right. Note that the titles tell us about the subject being discussed and the methodology. The headlines, which all have verbs, give the messages. Defining a message before writing is more useful than just writing a title because it gives direction and focus.

Title	Message
Mortality after *Staphylococcus aureus* bacteraemia in two hospitals in Oxfordshire, 1997–2003: cohort study	Spread of MRSA increases in hospitals
Health professionals' and service users' interpretation of screening test results: experimental study	Both screened and screeners misinterpret test results
Varicose veins and their management	Manage varicose veins with conventional surgery
Triggering radiation alarms after radioiodine treatment	Radiotherapy patients can trigger airport radiation alarms

Do not confuse the message with a title. We shall return to titles (briefly – because they should not take more than a minute to write!) in Chapter 8, but at this stage the point to stress is that you do not need to write a title yet, and doing so could positively hinder your progress over the next few weeks. A message will give you the direction you are going to take (*see* Figure 3.2); a title will normally indicate only which broad area you are to cover. Similarly, at this stage we do not want a question; we want the answer.

Choose the market

Once you have decided on your message, ask: 'In which journal do I intend to have it published?' This is another difficult question, and again many authors delay their decision until after they have written the article. Perhaps they hope that the solution will emerge as they move along the writing process, or that the finished paper will somehow be so good that every editor will be fighting to take it.

Nevertheless, there are resounding arguments for matching message to market at this early stage. You can make an informed decision, before you start committing time and energy, as to whether the publication you are considering is likely to publish an article of the type you are about to write. It is better to do this now than it is to discover, too late, that you have been writing an article that no one is likely to publish. Another advantage is that, once you have decided on the target journal, you will have evidence that will guide you as you go through the writing process, and will help you later as you come to discuss your work with your colleagues. Find a copy of the journal's *Instructions to authors* (*see* Figure 3.3) and read them carefully. Look out for past issues of your target journal so that you can see how that journal (and

FIGURE 3.3 Guidance to authors

All journals publish some kind of guidance to authors, ranging from sporadically published *Instructions to authors* to large series of web pages devoted to everything an author needs to know (and some things they probably don't). This guidance is valuable information, and prospective authors must study it closely and often, both while choosing a target journal and subsequently working on the manuscript. They should also bear in mind that this information has its limitations: it is what editors think they want rather than what they actually do, and it should not replace looking at, and analysing, the actual contents.

On one level this information will give precise instructions in important areas such as how to present the manuscript, where and how to send it, and so on. It will also deal with some of the issues that come with publication, such as copyright assignment and whether offprints are supplied. On a more subtle level it will give you a valuable flavour of the journal's personality and, presumably, that of the editor(s). Compare these two contrasting extracts:* apart from the specific instructions, what clues do they give about what each journal wants?

The *British Journal of Dermatology* (*BJD*) strives to publish the highest quality dermatological research. In so doing, the journal aims to advance understanding, management and treatment of skin disease and improve patient outcomes.

BJD invites submissions under a broad scope of topics relevant to clinical and experimental research and publishes original articles, reviews, concise communications, case reports and items of correspondence . . .

BJD is an official organ of the British Association of Dermatologists but attracts contributions from all countries in which sound research is carried out, and its circulation is equally international. The overriding criteria for publication are scientific merit, originality and interest to a multidisciplinary audience.

The *Journal of Investigative Dermatology* (*JID*) publishes reports describing original research on all aspects of cutaneous biology and skin disease . . .

Case reports or case series, unless they provide new biologic insights, are rarely appropriate for the Journal. Mutation reports of mutations in known genes with no new mechanistic data will not be considered . . .

Reports that primarily or exclusively concern a methodology, with the data documenting utility or feasibility, rather than providing new biologic insights, are discouraged, although exceptions to our policy of rejection may occasionally be made. Submissions reporting new methods in combination with mechanistic insights into the problem being investigated are, in contrast, most welcome.

*Taken from websites in April 2015.

FIGURE 3.4 Choosing a journal

Some of the important factors to be considered when choosing a journal are these:

- your goals – and the goals of others in your team
- the strength (and newsworthiness) of the message
- the robustness of the methods used
- evidence of a 'thread' or conversation on that topic within a journal
- a format that is clearly used by the journal
- links with the journal – so that you can get good 'market information'
- the status of the journal, as measured (allegedly) by impact factor.

its editor) likes their papers to look, and that information will prove invaluable in the weeks to come.

All this is obvious. In practice the problem is: how do you choose the target journal in the first place? (*See* Figure 3.4.) There is no easy answer. The message you wish to put across will be a useful starting point and should narrow the field considerably.

Another consideration is what you want to get out of publication. (Chapter 2 should have helped you with this.) If you want fame across the profession, aim for a general journal, such as *Nature*, *The Lancet*, the *BMJ* or *The New England Journal of Medicine*. If you seek promotion, go for those with the highest impact factors (*see* Figure 3.5). If you want to influence a small group of doctors only, choose the specialist journal they read.

You may wish to produce a shortlist of four or five journals. If you still find it difficult to choose, run a literature search. How much has each of them published about your subject in the past few years? You will find that journals, like their editors, show patterns of interest or 'threads' – preferences for dealing with certain topics and shunning others. This piece of market research should help you to make an informed decision, but if you still find it hard to decide, choose a journal you read and enjoy because, as a regular reader, you will be comfortable with its style and approach. Knowing someone connected with a journal can also help, not because they can pull strings (they usually can't and/or won't) but because they will be able to give you good 'market information'.

Do not be shy of ambition. If you want (or need) to be published in a top journal, study that journal closely.

FIGURE 3.5 The tyranny of the impact factor

Eugene Garfield's grand idea was that he could produce league tables of journals by counting the number of times each paper published in each journal was subsequently cited by other authors. This led to the impact factor, run by the Institute for Scientific Information and now operated by Thomson Scientific. Their annual publication *Journal Citation Reports* claims to provide a 'systematic, objective way to evaluate the world's leading journals and their impact and influence in the global research community'.

Various studies have shown that an impact factor can be affected by all kinds of actions, such as being reported in the mainstream press, accompanied by large numbers of sponsored reprints, or simply requests from editors to include references from their journals. Editors have also discovered that they can make major increases to their scores simply by rejigging their journals.

None of this would matter much had not civil servants and academic administrators adopted impact factors as a measure of 'quality'. Now researchers and clinicians need to publish in high impact publications for their promotions, and the groups they work in need to publish in high impact publications to secure funding. Pressure to publish has become pressure to publish in a high-ranked journal.

The problem this raises, particularly for those less experienced in this publication game, is what to do with a paper that, with all the goodwill in the world, will never be published in a high impact journal. This raises the interesting – albeit too late to ask once the work has been undertaken – question of why the work was done in the first place. One option is to send the paper to a high impact journal 'just in case'; however, this has all the logic of sending artichokes to someone who is looking for lemons. A second option is to shelve it quietly. This is demoralising, causes publication bias and is unethical. The third solution, which I wholeheartedly commend, is to seek publication in an appropriate journal, regardless of the fact that it may not have a high impact factor. It will be a useful learning experience, build confidence – and, more importantly, put pieces of knowledge that have been carefully teased out into the public domain, which is where they should be.

http://thomsonreuters.com/en.html

Some selected impact factors*

N Engl J Med	54.4
Nature	42.4
JAMA	30.0
BMJ	16.3
PLoS Med	14.0
Gut	13.3
Am J Gastroenterol	9.2
Pediatrics	5.3
Med Educ	3.6
J Paediatr Child Health (Australia/New Zealand)	1.2

*Taken from individual journal websites in April 2015.

Look at the articles in your specialty it has published recently. Can you provide, and support, a message of comparable quality? If so, there is no reason why you should not be able to become published, irrespective of your (current) place in the hierarchy.

The most important thing is to be rational. The question is not 'Where would I like to get published?' but 'Who is likely to publish me?'

Decide on the length

How long should your article be? The answer now becomes quite simple: it is what your target journal requires. You should find this covered in the journal's *Instructions to authors*, but you would do well to take some articles and count the paragraphs; these are a more manageable unit than words alone. The principle is that length is determined not by how much you wish to write, but by what the market will bear.

You will doubtless feel you need more space to do yourself justice; everyone does. Note the story (probably apocryphal, because I hear it attributed to different writers depending on which country I'm in) about the literary figure who wrote: 'I apologise for such a long letter; I didn't have time to write a short one.' It conveys an important truth: all writing can be shortened. It will make life harder for you, but easier for your reader.

Agree the deadlines

Having a plan of what to write, and for whom, won't give you the necessary momentum unless you put a deadline on it. The previous chapter stressed the importance of this.

But you should do more than set a deadline; set several. Writing and submitting a scientific article is a huge task, and unless you approach it with stealth and cunning, the nearer you get to it, the further away it will seem to move. Break this large task down into smaller ones, and turn this into a schedule (*see* Figure 3.6). Making sure you – and your colleagues – keep to it will be one of the most important ways you can work towards publication.

FIGURE 3.6 Sample schedule

Set the brief	1 January
Finish first draft	15 January
Send to co-authors	15 February
Back from co-authors	15 March
Send off	1 April

Agree on the co-authors

Writing is a personal activity. Someone has to do the solitary tasks like thinking, planning, writing, rewriting and arbitrating between opposing views. If you are the person who is doing all this, you have a sound moral case to be the first author. As such, you are in effect the team leader, and the responsibility of managing the project is yours. There are several things you can do to smooth the path to publication (*see* Figure 3.7).

Resist the notion of writing in committee. Committees are not suitable because the emphasis inevitably switches from pleasing the target reader to pleasing those forming the committee. You will need contributions from other members of the team, but it will be your responsibility to solicit them individually, make decisions about them and generally reconcile opposing views.

Whom should you name as your co-authors? Here there is not only potential conflict between you and your colleagues, but between you and your future editor.

FIGURE 3.7 How to get the most out of your writing team

- Set annual targets – and help people keep to them.
- Encourage people to persevere rather than criticise their early efforts.
- Do not act unethically (e.g. over authorship).
- Agree as much as you can before you start.
- Make sure writers are resourced (time to write, go on courses etc.).
- Give balanced feedback (not just a string of criticisms).
- Keep to deadlines.
- Reward success.

Editors over the years have discovered clear cases of abuse or 'ghost authorship', when people who had no right to share the credit have insisted that their names be included. They now take a tough line and say that authorship should be based only on 'substantial contributions' (*see* Figure 3.8). This does not impress those who see clearly that getting their name on a paper will considerably increase their chances of progressing in their careers. This is really a political question, not a writing one. First authors have to compromise, particularly if those who wish to be associated as co-authors are higher up the hierarchy. What you must guard against is having so many co-authors that your paper starts to look ridiculous, such as 12 authors reporting tests on three dogs. There comes a point where it could jeopardise your chances of publication.

One way of reducing the strain is to negotiate on all aspects of the question of authorship *before* you start the writing. Work out as far as possible who will be

FIGURE 3.8 The editors' view of authorship

According to the International Committee of Medical Journal Editors (ICMJE – formerly known as the Vancouver Group), an author must have made 'substantial intellectual contributions to a published study'.

Their statement gives the following criteria.

1. Substantial contributions to the conception or design of the work; or the acquisition, analysis, or interpretation of data for the work; AND
2. Drafting the work or revising it critically for important intellectual content; AND
3. Final approval of the version to be published; AND
4. Agreement to be accountable for all aspects of the work in ensuring that questions related to the accuracy or integrity of any part of the work are appropriately investigated and resolved.

The guidelines add: 'In addition to being accountable for the parts of the work he or she has done, an author should be able to identify which co-authors are responsible for specific other parts of the work. In addition, authors should have confidence in the integrity of the contributions of their co-authors. All those designated as authors should meet all four criteria for authorship, and all who meet the four criteria should be identified as authors.'

www.icmje.org

your co-authors, what the role of each of them will be and in what order their names will appear. This should eliminate some of the worst excesses. It should also ease the strain in the latter stages of the writing process,

when many hours can be wasted because the co-authors
– without realising it – are actually trying to write different papers with different messages. Before you go any
further, send them in writing a copy of the message you
propose, and ask if they agree.

Some people find setting the brief extremely difficult.
That's probably because, if done properly, it is difficult.
But time spent on setting a sensible brief, and, in particular, on deciding in advance what message you choose to
give (*see* Figure 3.9) will pay huge benefits later.

FIGURE 3.9 Setting the brief

Example A

Message:	A multinational trial of 2373 post-lunchtime amnesia sufferers has shown that Obecalp is more effective than the established treatment
Market:	*The Lancet*
Length:	2500 words
Deadline:	First draft by 13 July
Co-authors:	All those involved in the seven centres

Example B

Message:	Three out of seven patients with chronic post-lunchtime amnesia went into immediate remission after a diet of dandelion leaves and frankfurters
Market:	*Journal of the Society of Postprandial Pathologists*
Length:	1000 words
Deadline:	First draft by tomorrow week
Co-authors:	The medical student who first spotted it and the consultant you report to

CHECKPOINT

Before proceeding to Chapter 4, you should have a clear brief, with agreed written statements on the following:

1. the message (one simple idea, with verb)
2. the market
3. the length
4. the deadline
5. the co-authors.

You should also be familiar with your target journal's *Instructions to authors*.

4

Expand the brief

'The mess in my head is now a mess on a piece of paper.'

Gather your strength

This is a key moment. You may still be worrying that you have not made any progress, and that soon you are going to have to take the plunge and start writing. In fact, you are not merely over the worst, you have decided on the message and so have written your article. Admittedly, at this stage it consists of one idea and is 10–14 words long. But you have made the all-important decision on what precisely, when all else is cut away (or lost in the mists of the reader's memory), you wish your reader to understand. You have also made the vital decision on where you will publish. You have defined your product, and now all you have to do is flesh it out.

There are two ways of proceeding. The first is the 'clerical' approach. This means going through all the material, in no particular order, pulling out bits of data, tables and references, and allocating them to one of

papers, life is made relatively easy by the fact that there are four main questions to ask:

- Why did we start?
- What did we do?
- What did we find?
- What does it all mean?

Expand the spidergram

You will now be able to use this framework to expand on your message (*see* Figure 4.2). The principles are these.

- Take one question and start writing down points you will need to answer it.
- When you have run out of things to say on one line of questioning, go on to the next.
- Use one bit of information (one or two words) at a time.
- Work fast – and once you have put something down move forward; avoid crossings out.
- Everything should be linked back to the message with a line.
- Do not be afraid to link various words together.
- Avoid writing lists, or complete sentences.

Starting with the first question ('Why did we start?'), the following questions suggest themselves.

- What topic/subject are we looking at?
- What do we know about this?

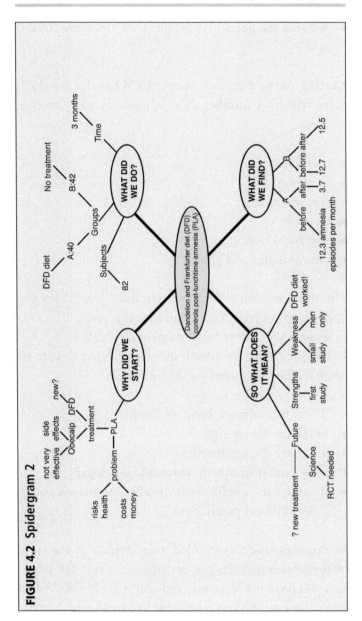

FIGURE 4.2 Spidergram 2

- What is the particular problem we are going to deal with?

Moving on to the next question ('What did we do?') there will be a number of sub-headings you can use, such as:

- subjects
- interventions
- measurements
- timeline
- statistical tests
- ethical issues and approval.

The third section ('What did we find?') provides the opportunity to record the results. Ideally, you will be able to divide these into a small number of bundles.

Finally, comes the fourth question: 'What does it all mean?' Here the questions might include:

- What, in summary, have we found?
- What are the strengths?
- What are the weaknesses?
- How does it fit in with current knowledge?
- What are the implications for science, current policy and/or clinical practice?

At this stage the tidy-minded often despair at the state of their spidergrams, but orderliness is not the issue. You will have made a start; and you will have started to move information out from your head and onto a piece of paper (or computer screen). Apart from guiding you through the deep sludge of writer's block, this will provide a bank of information and ideas from which you will be able to consolidate your article. Messy perhaps, but the fact that there are now words to look at means that you are in control.

There is another advantage. Everything on your spidergram should have a route back to the central message, and therefore be specifically related to it. You have begun the task of working out what is relevant to your message and what is not (however interesting it might be). What is important is not just what you have put in, but what your thought processes have led you to leave out.

Do not be too smug, however. You have not yet planned your article. What you have done is make selections from the mass of information you have in your head, and started to sort it. This will stand you in good stead when you get to the next phase, which is writing a linear plan.

---

❷ CHECKPOINT

Before proceeding to Chapter 5, you should have a large piece of paper containing the message – and the main things you will need to put into your article to support that message.

BOOKCHOICE: Thinking and sorting

Buzan T and Buzan B (2010) *The Mind Map Book: unlock your creativity, boost your memory, change your life*. BBC Active, Harlow.

If you like the idea of spidergrams then you will certainly enjoy looking at the work of Tony Buzan. He was the creator in the 1960s of mind mapping, which is now an international brand that he claims 'allows access to the vast thinking powerhouse of the brain'.

Buzan had become disenchanted with the monotony of (monotone) lists and decided that harnessing the structures of the brain to unleash imagination and association could improve memory and creativity. Like the spidergrams shown in this chapter, his mind maps consist of ideas radiating out from a single thought or message. But Buzan takes this further by advocating pictures, colours and curved lines. The mind maps that follow, he says, allow the creator to have an overview, make choices, collect data, solve problems – and have fun. He describes them as 'the ultimate thinking tool'.

This book is one of many that Buzan has written on the topic. It is lavishly produced, with plenty of examples of his brainchild in action. It covers mind maps for self-analysis, study skills, meetings and presentations – and has a final section on electronic mind maps. There are some telling examples. I particularly liked the one of the star pupil whose grades started to fall at the same time as her note-taking became more and more elaborate;

mind mapping reversed the trend. The technique is not for everyone, but those who do use it find it invaluable.

www.thinkbuzan.com

5

Make a plan, or four

'Drawing a creative (non-linear) pattern is often useful for gathering ideas and as a start to the planning stage; converting this to a logical linear structure may be more difficult.'

Understanding structure 1: the paragraph

Your head should be bursting with details of the work you have done. You now need to start making some decisions – but before you do so it is helpful to understand some of the elements of structure.

One of the common ways of talking about writing is in terms of total number of words. This is not helpful. The problem is not the quantity of words, but how you group them together and order them.

A more fruitful way forward is to think of the paragraph as the main unit. Each paragraph is a block of type that stands alone, and therefore it is sensible to assume that each covers a particular area. As for construction, the trick is to realise that there are two types of sentences. Go through a piece of text and underline or highlight the key sentences so that you are left with a much smaller version than your original text. This has divided your sentences into two types. The 'key' sentences – those that you have underlined – move the argument forward. The 'supporting' sentences – those not underlined – illustrate and support your arguments.

Should the 'key' sentences appear at the beginning of each paragraph or at the end? Scientists tend to structure all their writing in the style of IMRAD. Thus:

> *It is well documented that fires in nightclubs are a major hazard* [Introduction]. *Last night I went to a fire that took place in a nightclub in the middle of town and spoke to the senior fire officer* [Methods]. *He told me that 87 people perished* [Results]. *It is believed that fewer people would have died had the fire exits not been locked* [Discussion].

The alternative is to start with the most important piece of information, then elaborate, explain and, if necessary, prove. This is commonly used by professional communicators, who call it (probably inaccurately from the mathematical point of view) the 'inverted triangle'. Thus:

> *Eighty-seven people have perished in a fire where all the emergency exits were locked. It happened in a nightclub in the centre of town shortly after*

*midnight last night. The number of deaths was
confirmed by the senior fire officer at the scene.*

Your paragraphs will work well, and keep the reader
interested, if you write them so that they become in effect
a series of inverted triangles. Put the key sentence at the
beginning of the paragraph, as, for instance:

We then selected the patients . . .

*Once we had selected the patients we gave them
a battery of tests . . .*

*There are three reasons why our findings are of
interest . . .*

Then you can add sentences that support and elaborate
these. This has important implications for the planning
of an article. If you can take out all but the key sentences
after you have written, obviously you can plan by deciding what these key sentences will cover.

Understanding structure 2: the scientific paper

Not long after the publication of the first edition of this
book I hit on an idea that I hoped would make it easier
to get across to beginning writers the importance of
structure. I engaged a researcher to sit in a library and
do various boring tasks, such as counting up the number of paragraphs in each of 300 different articles (*see*

FIGURE 5.1 Mean number of paragraphs per section in six different journals

	Introduction	Methods	Results	Discussion
N Engl J Med	2.6 (±1.1)	9.2 (±3.3)	8.9 (±3.8)	6.9 (±1.8)
*Lancet**	2.6 (±1.3)	7.6 (±3.6)	6.1 (±2.9)	7.0 (±2.6)
*BMJ**	2.3 (±0.9)	6.0 (±3.7)	5.9 (±3.1)	7.4 (±2.8)
J Pediatr	2.6 (±1.1)	6.7 (±3.4)	7.0 (±3.9)	7.3 (±2.8)
Pediatr Res	3.0 (±1.3)	9.6 (±3.8)	6.3 (±2.9)	8.5 (±3.4)
*Arch Dis Child**	2.7 (±1.3)	6.5 (±4.0)	6.1 (±4.0)	6.9 (±2.8)

Numbers in parentheses are the standard deviations.

*European-based journals.

Source: 50 consecutive articles from 1 June 1997. Full details available on www.timalbert.co.uk

Figure 5.1). Using these figures we were able to come up with the following 'typical' structure of a scientific paper.

- Introduction – 2 paragraphs
- Methods – 7 paragraphs
- Results – 7 paragraphs
- Discussion – 6 paragraphs

This can be shown as a diagram (*see* Figure 5.2). Each (inverted) triangle represents a paragraph. The four arrows represent another pattern that emerged: four key sentences appearing at these points in many of the manuscripts we looked at. This clearly can be used as a template for many scientific papers, though there are

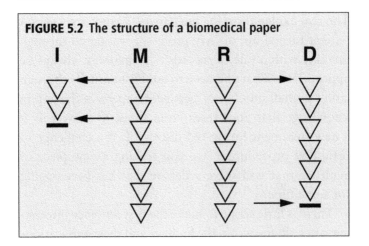

FIGURE 5.2 The structure of a biomedical paper

exceptions (qualitative studies, for instance, are more likely to have a structure along the lines of 2-2-14-6).

The work was done nearly 20 years ago and as far as I know has not been replicated. Since then the shape and length of papers have diversified dramatically, mainly because electronic publishing means that the length of papers is no longer influenced by the cost of paper production. But the main value of this research is not so much in showing the exact pattern, but in showing that this pattern can be measured. Before writing a plan, therefore, take out some recent copies of your target journal and find the pattern. (You will be surprised by how often, still, the 2-7-7-6 pattern recurs.)

This is market research, and will appear again later in these pages.

Introduction

This section answers the question: 'Why did we start?'

The real explanation for the paper ('We got a grant', 'A patient turned up' or 'My professor wandered through one day with a pile of records . . .') may not always be appropriate. What you need to establish, usually through citing a small number of pertinent papers, is the gap in knowledge that your research is about to answer. Is it a new treatment for an old disease? Is it a challenge to orthodox procedures? Are you seeking a new piece of evidence that will solve a debate that has been raging for some time?

There is little scope to make the first sentence interesting: after all, the work, the findings and their implications all have to appear elsewhere. This is probably why most authors follow one of a small number of stock openings. Most give a brief lesson on the subject that is to be embarked upon (the 'seminar approach', *see* Figure 5.3):

FIGURE 5.3 Types of first sentence in six different journals

	Seminar	Alarmist	MDR
N Engl J Med	45	2	3
*Lancet**	34	10	6
*BMJ**	37	4	9
J Pediatr	47	2	1
Pediatr Res	44	3	3
*Arch Dis Child**	43	4	3

*European-based journals.
Source: 50 consecutive articles from 1 June 1997.

> *Post-lunchtime amnesia in hospital doctors is characterised by a severe loss of memory 1 hour after consuming a meal of more than 87.3 calories taken between 12.10 and 1.45.*

An alternative, favoured by *The Lancet*, is to emphasise the gravity of the condition ('alarmist approach'):

> *Post-lunchtime amnesia kills 3000 people a year in UK hospitals.*

A third technique is to refer to a controversy ('much discussion recently' [MDR] approach):

> *There has been much discussion recently about the incidence and importance of post-lunchtime amnesia in hospital doctors.*

The Introduction becomes straightforward. It usually starts with a sentence focusing on the topic, then has five/ six sentences elaborating on this. The second paragraph starts with the particular problem; for example:

> *Until now there has been no successful treatment for post-lunchtime amnesia.*

After elaborating it will go on to the second key sentence of the article (the last sentence of the Introduction) which will tell the reader what the authors did:

We therefore undertook a multicentre randomised trial to see whether Obecalp had any effect on post-lunchtime amnesia.

The emergence of this key paragraph/sentence at the end of the Introduction is an interesting development. It could be used as an opening sentence for either the Introduction or the Discussion, but in its present form it acts as a hinge between the two sections.

Methods

This section answers the question: 'What did we do?'

It expands on the information just given in the final paragraph of the Introduction. It should give readers enough information to enable them to evaluate, and in theory to replicate, the work. It should also explain the statistical methods and make it clear that ethical guidelines were followed.

As a general principle, this section tells the story of what the authors did. Usually the best way to organise this will be in a logical framework of time.

Results

Again use a small number of bundles. These will tell the story of the main findings (not every detail of what you found – those will be in the tables, which we will deal with later).

Discussion

The common wisdom here is that this section is extremely difficult. Analysis suggests that it need not be. As before we analysed the two key sentences, and found a clear pattern.

The first sentence should state clearly in summary what you found. For instance:

Our study showed that Obecalp was effective . . .

We looked at three different last sentences (*see* Figure 5.4). One type had the 'More research is indicated' ending which happily is less common than is normally thought (after all it is a totally inconclusive conclusion).

The effectiveness of this intervention must be treated cautiously and requires verification in further experimental trials.

The second was the 'Perhaps possibly':

This might provide a basis for future treatment, or it might not.

FIGURE 5.4 Types of last sentence in six different journals

	Another puzzle solved	Perhaps possibly	More research is indicated
N Engl J Med	27	17	6
Lancet*	19	21	10
BMJ*	22	16	12
J Pediatr	26	16	8
Pediatr Res	20	20	10
Arch Dis Child*	27	10	13

*European-based journals.

The third was the 'Another puzzle solved' (aka the message).

> *This study provides evidence that we now have a good basis for future treatment.*

Quite clearly the last is the best alternative. What it means is that you are ending on your message, and this gives a clear structure to the narrative.

The paragraphs in between should not pose too much difficulty if taken logically. There are various things to do:

- explain the strengths of the research/paper
- explain the limitations
- explain how the paper fits into the context of previous work
- suggest the implications of the research for (a) future research, (b) future policy and/or (c) clinical practice.

Choose one paragraph for each point (perhaps more under exceptional circumstances) and you are almost there.

Writing the plan

Armed with this knowledge, writing the plan should be easy. What you are looking for is a road map that will identify what you will be saying in each paragraph. You might also wish to put down roughly what you will want each of your four key sentences to say (*see* Figure 5.5).

FIGURE 5.5 The four key sentences

Introduction first sentence: what we looked at
Introduction last sentence: what we did
Discussion first sentence: what we found
Discussion last sentence: what it means – THE MESSAGE!

The important thing is to keep the plan brief. The process of planning should take no longer than a few minutes. The purpose of this stage is to build the main branches of your tree – in other words, chart the main headings of your argument (*see* Figure 5.6). If you do not keep away from the details at this stage they will swamp you.

CHECKPOINT

At the end of this chapter you should have a simple plan for each of the four sections: Introduction, Methods, Results and Discussion.

FIGURE 5.6 A plan

Introduction

⟶ <u>Post-lunchtime amnesia is big problem.</u>
▽ Problem – elaborate
▽ Prevalence?
⟶ <u>We did questionnaire to find out how big.</u>

Methods

▽ Ethics
▽ Funding
▽ Questionnaire design
▽ Questionnaire admin
▽ Sample
▽ Exclusions
▽ Statistical analyses

Results

▽ Prevalence
▽ Surgeons vs physicians
▽ Seniors vs juniors
▽ Doctors vs nurses
▽ Male vs female
▽ Relationship to medical school
▽ Regional variations

Discussion

⟶ <u>We found it was a big, big problem!</u>
▽ Elaborate on problem
▽ Weaknesses?
▽ Strengths?
▽ How it fits in with literature
▽ Implications for research
▽ Implications for policy/treatment
⟶ <u>We need to act immediately to prevent post-lunchtime amnesia</u>

6

Write the first draft

'I was surprised at how much I could write in 10 minutes. This paper has sat unwritten for two years and I hope is now under way.'

Conquer the fear of writing . . .

The next part of the process is to start the actual writing. This should be fun, but seems to traumatise most people. They go to severe lengths to avoid it, and use various strategies such as hunting references, making coffee, telephoning unloved relatives or sitting for hours in front of a blank screen, blankly.

I blame the teachers, who have so brainwashed us that we cannot undertake a writing task without believing that it is an examination. But writing for a journal is not that kind of test. What is being judged is not what writers have happened to learn (or remember), but the particular contribution to knowledge that they are describing. It is not a time trial and what is important is not the first draft but the final version.

Understanding this should help to make this part of the writing process much less frightening. Putting the words down on paper becomes not an end point, but a beginning. This should be a time of creativity, not criticism (*see* Bookchoice, p. 69). If you have done the preparatory thinking, all the information and arguments are already lodged in your head; you now have to unlock them. What you write will not be perfect, but at this stage it doesn't matter.

Get ready to write

You need three things only for the writing process: a clear plan, a suitable writing implement, and peace and quiet.

A clear plan

Take only your plan with you into this stage. Do not surround yourself with all the raw material, such as tables and references and longhand notes of seminar papers. It matters little at this stage whether your experiment killed 43 rats or 47; you will know that, since there were only 50, the trend was to die. Go for the flow; you can add the details later.

Incidentally, if you write your first draft in this way you will find it impossible to plagiarise!

A suitable writing implement

Most people write directly into a word processor of some kind. This can be fast and enjoyable, but there are two main problems. First, you may be tempted to go back and fiddle with words and phrases. Second, you may be tempted to go back and fiddle with whole paragraphs.

You need to resist such temptations as much as possible; if you really find it difficult try turning off the screen!

Some writers feel that using a dictating machine is cheating, but it has the advantage that you can swiftly put down a first draft. If you have someone who can then transcribe it for you, this is a painless way to start. You will be speaking aloud, and so are more likely to use the rhythms and vocabulary of oral speech (which is much easier to unravel than that which presently goes under the title of Proper Scientific Writing). Unfortunately, it can be too easy to get carried away with the sound of your own voice. If you choose this option, make sure that you have your plan in front of you while you are dictating.

Others prefer more traditional methods, such as a pen or pencil. These are relatively slow (and perhaps painful), but you can still do 30–40 words a minute if you write without stopping. Some swear that a fountain pen gives them the right speed. Others insist on a pencil with an eraser but, to stop you fiddling rather than writing, I would recommend cutting off the eraser.

Peace and quiet

Many people say that finding time is the major problem. They are extremely busy people (parents, lovers, doctors, scientists, model aeroplane society secretaries), and even when they manage to find time, either at home or at work, other people constantly interrupt them.

The answer is not to see when you can block off 2–3 hours of uninterrupted time; that is almost impossible these days. Instead try to snatch 20 minutes a day. For reasons that I am about to explain, that should be enough to write about 500 words. Four such snatches, and you will have completed the first draft of the paper. This is a controversial assertion, but, if true, think of how it will revolutionise your life. (As supporting evidence I can state that in 20 minutes I managed to write the first 720 words of the first draft of this chapter.)

Go with the flow

The key is to be creative, not critical, and to turn the first draft from a penance into a festival. It should be fun.

At this stage you need big ideas and logical flow. You are the expert on the subject you have chosen. You also have a plan to remind you of the steps you have decided to take. Flesh these out: your goal is to end up with the outline of each section. There will almost certainly be gaps, but you can fill these later.

So, when you start to write, write down the first sentence immediately. If it isn't the perfect opening sentence (and it is unlikely that it will be) start with the second sentence. Or go back and take a run at the start with sentences that can easily be dismantled later, such as:

I am about to sit here for 20 minutes and write about the wonderful experiment I have just completed. What we did was . . .

When you have finished one sentence, go on to the next. When you have finished that one, go on again. And so on. Do not under any circumstances look back.

Use your natural language. Do not try to imitate the

style of your chosen journal at this stage. Do not try to impress your professor. Instead, imagine that you are speaking to an informed colleague over a beer or coffee. Use the language with which you are most comfortable and you will probably find that it will end up much clearer than if you were consciously constructing individual sentences for publication. (You may have to translate this later into the dull style favoured by your target journal, but that will be straightforward.)

If your first language is not English, consider writing the first draft in your own language. At this stage we are talking about thought processes; an appropriate language can easily come later.

Whatever language you choose, by the end of 20 minutes or so (and again you may wish to put a timer on) you will have made considerable progress. You will have some words on paper and those words will have taken a shape.

Some people will never believe that writing in short bursts will solve their problems. They tend to be those who, as soon as they have written one sentence, will go back and worry about it. They constantly fiddle with the meaning, checking whether the references are exactly right, or looking up obscure points of punctuation in a heavy tome on grammar. Let them enjoy this process if they want – but it will reduce rather than increase their chances of getting published.

Write each section in turn

I know that many people recommend that you should start with the Methods section on the grounds that this is an easy place to start. But I recommend writing the sections in the order in which they will be read. This seems to be a logical way of doing things, and enables the writer to keep focused.

Overcome writer's block

From time to time you will find it impossible to get going, or you will simply dry up. This is commonly called 'writer's block'. It can be nature's way of telling you that you are bored – in which case the solution is simple: do something else. Most people have their times when they seem to write best: work out when yours is. If you cannot force the pace at other times, don't feel guilty. Stop.

However, writer's block can also be your subconscious mind's way of telling you that your writing has lost its way. In this case it is also time to call a temporary halt. You might wish to talk to a colleague. If that fails to work, walk away from the article, take a good rest and then think out the brief again. You should have already spotted if you were persevering with the unpublishable, so the worst possible scenario is that you will have to start again from scratch. Since you have done most of the research, that will take much less time than you will think, and certainly will cost much less time than if you continue on your fruitless task.

> **CHECKPOINT**
>
> Before proceeding to Chapter 7, you should have four rough drafts of the Introduction, Methods, Results and Discussion.

BOOKCHOICE: Writing without pain and guilt

Klauser HA (1987) *Writing on Both Sides of the Brain: breakthrough techniques for people who write.* HarperCollins, San Francisco.

This is a gem of a book, despite its somewhat gushing tone. It is nearly 30 years old now, and no longer listed at bookshops. But it was a great influence on my courses and I have not yet found another book that deals so well with the various *processes* involved in writing.

It is full of sensible advice that should leave you motivated to start – and, more importantly, finish – your next writing task. The key notion is the division of our brains into two sides, and with it the division of writing into two functions – the critical and the creative (or what Klauser calls, after characters in *The Tempest*, Caliban and Ariel). We need both – but not at the same time.

From this comes a number of excellent ideas:

- start a log so that you can write about your writing – what you are achieving and where your problems lie
- consider your rumination time an essential part of writing

- when writing and thinking about writing, try to go that extra bit further (what she calls 'hitting the wall')
- write without judging what you are writing (i.e. give yourself 'permission to write garbage')
- start writing first thing in the morning . . .

As Klauser says, the book is for you 'if you are tired of putting off the writing that needs to be done, if you believe that you have an idea locked up inside of you that you lack the confidence to share in writing, if you are holding yourself back from getting a promotion because you are not doing the writing that your chosen profession calls for . . .' If you see the book in a second-hand shop, snap it up.

7

Rewrite your draft

'I now have concrete pointers on which I can evaluate my own work.'

Now comes the pain . . .

Once you have finished your first draft, walk away from it. Leave it for a time: some people say for a few days, but this may not always be practicable. The important thing is to put some distance between you and it, so you will be able to approach it with some objectivity, and not see it as a part of your soul that others tamper with at their peril.

When you return, brace yourself for some hard work. Some people complain that they spend too much time rewriting. I suspect that they are still hung up on the feeling that they must get it right first time. The real test of a piece of writing is not how quickly it was written, but whether it works for the target audience. To complain that you have a writing problem because you took 12 or so drafts for an article that was published in *Nature* is missing the point. As with all products, the secret to success is hard work; if something looks polished, the chances are that someone has spent a lot of time doing the polishing.

Sometimes things do go wrong, however, and you find that you are getting nowhere: the last eight drafts, for instance, may have taken you back to where you started some weeks ago. There are ways of limiting such disasters. First, keep to your deadlines, which will cut down your inclination to fiddle for the sake of fiddling. Second, for at least some of the time, rewrite on hard copy rather than on screen, which again will reduce the opportunity for uncontrolled fiddling. Third, have clear in your own mind the criteria you will use for judging what you have written, and how you will go about applying them.

As a start, I recommend dividing this process into two: macroediting and microediting.

Macroediting

Print out your first draft and read it privately. You do not need a pencil at this stage. Try not to worry if the words are misspelt (as some of them certainly will be) or if some of the details are still missing. Read the article through quickly to get some impression of how it looks now that it has moved from your head onto a piece of paper. Then start asking yourself the difficult questions.

Is there a clear message?

What was the message you chose to write about? Where does it appear? Will it be clear to your target audience (i.e. the editor)? Is what you set out to say the same as what you have written? Or have some changes of emphasis crept in? Is your message clearly positioned in the last sentence of the Discussion? Now that the message is in black and white, does it still look worth saying?

These are central questions. No matter how polished your prose, publication is unlikely unless you are saying something worthwhile – a clear and interesting message clearly stated where the audience wants to find it. By now you should have that clear and interesting message; after all you spent plenty of time working on it in the earlier stages. The main thing is to make sure it hasn't got lost in the excitement of writing!

Do you prove your message?

Given that you have a clear message in place, do you prove it? Is the evidence clearly stated and well supported? If you were your own worst enemy (or competing against yourself for a job) how would you criticise the article? If there are weaknesses in the defences, how can you strengthen them? If you can't, make sure they are covered (nicely) in the paragraph on limitations.

Is it right for the market you have chosen?

This question is usually straightforward. Again, you will have spent some time in the preparatory stages matching message to market, and it is unlikely that the process of writing the first draft will have caused you to change your mind.

Is the tone appropriate?

Most journals cultivate a particular tone (often a rather

pompous one, it must be said, but that's another story). But this is easy to measure, using one of the various 'readability' scores (*see* Figure 7.1). Make sure that your submission conforms.

Is the structure appropriate and reader friendly?

First remind yourself of the typical structure (i.e. paragraphs per section) of your target journal. Let's say that comes to 2-7-7-6. Then count up the number of paragraphs per section in your draft. If there is some minor variation, with reasons that you can identify, don't worry. But if there are gross variations, you may need to do some restructuring. A pattern of 7-7-7-3, for instance, might suggest that you need to move some information from the Introduction to the Discussion. A pattern of 2-18-7-6 might suggest that you consider putting some of your methods into an appendix. A pattern of 2-7-16-6 might suggest that you have two papers. And a pattern of 2-7-7-3 might suggest that you turn this into a short paper before the editor suggests that you do so.

Next carry out the 'yellow marker' test (*see* Figure 7.2). Do your key sentences come at the start of each paragraph? Do your paragraphs follow on from each other in a sensible fashion? If the test identifies any problems take remedial action.

Now turn to the four key sentences in an exercise I call 'storyboarding'. Write down the first and last sentences of the Introduction and the first and last sentences of the Discussion (*see* Figure 5.5). Is the first of these sentences a mini-seminar (a general introduction to the

FIGURE 7.1 Gunning Fog Score[7]

There are several tests of whether a piece of writing is likely to be easily readable or not, and the one I favour was the one devised in the early 1940s by Professor Gunning in the USA. It is based on the assumption that the longer the words and the longer the sentences, then the harder a piece of writing is likely to be.

The index is calculated using the following steps.

1. Count up a passage of about 100 words, ending in a full stop.
2. Calculate the average sentence length by dividing 100 by the number of sentences.
3. Count the number of long words, defined as words of three syllables or more, but excluding:
   - two-syllable verbs that become three by 'ed' or 'ing' (e.g. committed, committing)
   - proper nouns, like Winchester or Canterbury or Germany or Italy
   - two common short words used together, such as photocopy
   - jargon that readers will know (be very careful with interpreting this).
4. Add the average sentence length to the number of long words.
5. Multiply by 0.4. That is the reading score.

Typical scores: Airport novel 6; tabloid newspapers 8–10; middlebrow newspapers 10–12; serious newspapers 12–14; medical journals 14–16; insurance company small print 20.

Examples

'In conclusion, our data support the hypothesis that

non-steroidal anti-inflammatory drug use protects against the development of colorectal neoplasia./ The strength of the association is similar to that found in the three other epidemiological studies in which non-steroidal anti-inflammatory drug use has been associated with a halving of the risk of colorectal cancer./ Studies are now needed to confirm these findings, to determine how non-steroidal anti-inflammatory drugs might act, and particularly to see if non-steroidal anti-inflammatory drugs can prevent the recurrence of adenoma or even cause sporadic adenomas to regress.' – BMJ

'Aspirin, once seen as a humble household remedy for headaches, may also protect against bowel cancer as well as helping with arthritis and reducing the risk of heart disease and strokes, says a report in the BMJ today./ The study was done by Dr Richard Logan and colleagues from the University of Nottingham Medical School./ They say that those who took aspirin or other non-steroidal anti-inflammatory drugs (NSAIDs) had half the risk of developing the pre-cancerous lumps which go onto become bowel cancer as non-takers./ In some cases the dose was as low as half an aspirin a day.' – Guardian

		BMJ	Guardian
1	Number of sentences	3	4
2	Average sentence length	33	25
3	Long words	24	9
4	2 + 3	57	34
5	Fog Score (× 0.4)	22.8	13.6

The index does not predict good writing, so artificially manipulating it won't automatically turn something unreadable into something that is easy to read. But it does seem to correlate with readable writing.

There is no such thing as a 'good' or 'bad' score in isolation. The most important thing is that the score of your text should match the score of your market. When writing for a particular journal, take a selection of articles and do a Fog Score on them. Yours should be a comparable score.

The test can also give useful information if there is a particular writing problem. For instance, one student was sent on one of my courses on the grounds that she was a bad writer. Doing the test on her writing and on the writing of her professor showed that she was writing to a score of 12 (quite reasonable) while the professor favoured a tortuous style of 18.

FIGURE 7.2 The yellow marker test

The 'yellow marker' test can identify the underlying structure of an article. Go through with a marker pen and highlight those sentences that you feel are absolutely essential. This should leave you with a much shorter but still understandable version. This should show you the 'key' and 'supporting' sentences – plus the underlying structure of the writing.

Look at where these sentences fall. If most of the highlighted sentences come at the beginning of each paragraph, you will have a solid and easy-to-follow structure. If you have paragraphs with no sentences highlighted, ask: 'Is that paragraph necessary?' If you have highlighted several sentences together, ask: 'Am I risking information overload?' If the highlighted sentence is buried in the middle of a paragraph, ask: 'Would it work better at the beginning?'

topic)? Is the second a broad statement of what you did? Is the third a broad description of your findings? And is the fourth a summary of what it means – in other words the message?

The storyboard should allow you to see whether you are telling a simple and coherent story:

Post-lunchtime amnesia is a problem . . . we did a survey . . . we found prevalence high . . . we need to do something.

It should not go off in unexpected directions, as in:

The doctor–patient interface is very important . . . we looked at what food hospitals serve . . . we found high prevalence of post-lunchtime amnesia . . . afternoon appointments should start later.

Once you are satisfied that the four sentences tell your story, go back to the first one: is it as sharp as it could be (*see* Figure 7.3)?

These macroediting questions are important. But many people neglect them, probably because it is a lot easier to move commas around or repeat the rules of long-gone grammar teachers. Be patient: once you have asked the big questions – and have provided adequate solutions – you can start playing with the details.

FIGURE 7.3 First six words test

Conventions of a scientific paper dictate that the first sentence gives the background to the 'story' rather than (as with mainstream journalism) the essence of that story. But within that constraint there is plenty of scope for making the first sentence more – or less – interesting.

You can test your own first sentence by counting out the first six words of your article. Why six words? It is to some extent arbitrary, but it gives the writer enough time to establish the subject and the reader enough words to establish if he or she will be interested. And it can be revealing, as shown in the following examples.

In several articles the first six words were empty words or padding – 'throat clearing' – that could profitably have been removed, such as:

It has been suggested that up . . .
It is generally accepted that the . . .
There has been much discussion recently . . .

Other sentences started with precise – but not important – details that would have been better left until later in the sentence, or paragraph:

On 24 and 25 June 2012 . . .
Since the late 1990s most public . . .
In the Netherlands the prevention of . . .

The following sentences, on the other hand, work much better. The subject of the sentence (and of the article itself) is early in the first sentence. They are therefore far more likely to grab and keep the interest:

Wine has an ancient reputation for . . .
Insulin-dependent diabetes develops on the . . .
Oral contraceptives have been linked with . . .
Most low birthweight babies have a . . .

Microediting

Omssions and errors

Now is the time to check your facts and add any missing ones. Go back to your 'raw material'. Was it 1349 or 1347 rats that died? Have you allowed a decimal point to move? (When talking about doses, for instance, this could literally be a fatal mistake.) Are all your numbers consistent? 7 + 5 + 12 does not come to 23, and 7 is 29.1% not 21.9% of that total. Was that important paper published by Smith, Smith and Jones on page 1147, or by Smith, Jones and Smith on page 1174?

Now is the time to be obsessive. Nothing will ruin your hard work more quickly and more effectively than the discovery, after publication, that there are several inaccuracies that could (or should) have been avoided.

Many journals provide checklists: this is the time to read them, and make sure that you comply.

Spelling and grammar

Most computers have a spell check. Use it. It will take minutes rather than hours, and you will almost certainly pick up one or two misspellings that you have not and (since you wrote them in the first place) probably will not spot. (For instance, did you notice the missing 'i' from 'omissions' in the earlier heading?) Spell checks, however, are fallible and will not alert you to good words in the wrong place, as in: *Two bee whore knot two bee* . . .

Grammar will give you many more problems, mainly because it has become a battleground for those who wish to score points and assert that they have had a better education. These people cite certain 'rules' that they learnt at school, and scream with delight whenever you break one of them. In general these rules are limited to the following:

1. do not start a sentence with And or But
2. do not split an infinitive
3. do not end with a preposition.

Unfortunately for these critics, most contemporary authorities say that these rules are now outdated. My treasured copy of *The Good English Guide* says this about split infinitives: 'If you don't want to upset any-one, you will avoid split infinitives. If you care more about writing good clear English, you will be prepared *to fearlessly split* any infinitive to allow words to fall naturally.'[8] Gowers was clear about starting a sentence with 'But': 'The idea is now dead.'[9]

We should not slavishly follow rules that have passed their natural shelf life. Nor should we feel inferior in education or ability if we didn't happen to attend a school that gave formal grammar classes. Nevertheless, we do need to follow the main grammatical rules if we wish to make ourselves understood. One solution is to use one of the many software packages that have grammar checks. Unfortunately these take a long time to run, and are of limited value if, for instance, they keep telling you that you are breaking a rule of which you are completely ignorant.

My own recommendations are:

1. invest in a good but short book (*see* Bookchoice, p. 89)
2. find a friend who knows about grammar (but preferably a stylist rather than a pedant)
3. read your own words carefully, and apply common sense.

You do not need to know the definition of a 'dangling modifier' to realise that there is something wrong with the following:

> *Having vomited all night, the doctor visited the patient with a bowl.*

Style: in theory

There is a distinguished tradition in English writing – from George Orwell and Somerset Maugham to Philip Howard and Keith Waterhouse – that firmly equates style with energy, clarity and simplicity. Editors of scientific journals adhere to these principles, as do those who write on scientific writing.

Nearly 80 years ago *The Lancet* published the following advice: 'Every sentence should be as simple as possible: apart from technical terms it should be intelligible at a first reading to any educated person. The pompous circumlocution often thought appropriate to scientific publications is an enemy to clear thinking and an obstacle to the spread of information among busy practitioners.'[10] In 1996 the authors of *Successful Scientific Writing* expressed a similar view: 'A scientific paper should hold the attention of its readers by the importance of its content, not by its literary presentation. For this reason, the simplest writing style is usually best. This does not mean that you should avoid technical words . . . What it does mean is that you should not include verbose words and phrases in a vain attempt to impress the reader with your intellect and scientific status.'[11]

Every year more books are published with similar sentiments, accompanied by long lists of how to acquire a good style. More are coming out as I write. In view of the fact that the publication of these instructions has had absolutely no effect so far, I would suggest that you should merely ask the following three questions. Dealing with them sensibly will improve your prose considerably.

1 Are any sentences too long? One of the most common ways in which writing goes wrong is when sentences become complex and overloaded. The Fog Test (*see* Figure 7.1) suggests that we should be getting four to five sentences every 100 words (which is not the same as saying all sentences should be 20–25 words long). If the length starts to rise towards and beyond 30 words, you could be heading for trouble.

One common fault is to start with a subordinate phrase or clause, or even two:

> *Since long-term survival seems to be similar after initial resuscitation, whether this occurs in or outside hospital (81% over 2 years), any improvement in the success of cardiopulmonary resuscitation outside hospital would be beneficial.*

Then there is the reverse hamburger of a sentence, where the meat is ruined by a soggy mass in the middle:

> *The development of vaccines against infection with hepatitis B, initially by purification of the virus surface protein from the plasma of carriers and more recently via its synthesis in yeast by using recombinant DNA technology, has enabled the chain of infection to be broken.*

Finally comes the overload:

> *When only gastroscopy requests meant to exclude malignancy are tolerated, an adequate prediction model for peptic ulcer, or using a serologic test for further selection, not only helps by reducing the number of gastroscopy requests for other reasons, but also might support the decision to prescribe H_2-receptor antagonists before ordering further diagnostic tests.*

In this case, the best thing is to start again, perhaps by trying to tell a colleague what you are trying to say. You might find it helpful to do this in the pub, or a similar social setting.

2 Are there any passives that would be better in the active voice? The best way to start a sentence in English is with the subject:

> *As concern about the impact of current economic conditions on public health was shown by a*

substantial number of epidemiologists, the main activity was still investigation of medical priorities in the light of a background of decreasing wealth and employment opportunities.

can become:

Many epidemiologists were worried about the impact of current economic conditions on public health. They therefore concentrated on investigating medical priorities amid a background of decreasing wealth and employment opportunities.

Richard Smith, former editor of the *BMJ*, is clear which version he would prefer: 'The tragedy of scientific writing is that whole generations of young people who started writing:

The cat sat on the mat and *Mummy is eating an orange*

have been forced to write:

The mat is sat on by the cat

and:

The orange is being eaten by Mummy

because it is more scientific. Nobody knows why it is supposed to be more scientific, but I imagine that it has something to do with the objectivity of science.'[12]

What he means is many scientists still insist that the

passive is more objective, a concept that I find difficult to accept.

The passive is preferred

illustrates the main problem: who is doing the preferring? The writer? The writer and his friends? Most people? A lot of people? There is a lack of clarity, which is absent in the following active versions:

I prefer the active, or *Many scientists who were at school before the 1960s prefer the passive.*

3 Are there long words that could be replaced with shorter ones? Long words are not a sign of cleverness. Scientists may feel they have to use 'approximately' rather than 'about', but in no sense is the latter less scientific. Taken to extremes, a sentence such as:

We would not have enough hospital beds if there were a major asthma epidemic.

becomes:

Once a designated hospital is saturated, patients are diverted to supporting hospitals; but this option would not be available in a large epidemic of asthma if all hospitals in an area were affected.

The answer is straightforward: be vigilant. To help in this task I have a list of 10 commonly used pompous words and phrases, with their shorter alternatives (*see* Figures 7.4 and 7.5). Eliminating these would be a start.

FIGURE 7.4 Ten pompous words to avoid and suggested alternatives

additional	more
approximately	about
assistance	help
commencement	start
elevated	raised, higher
frequently	often
following	after
participate	take part
possesses	has
proliferation	spread

FIGURE 7.5 Ten pompous phrases to avoid and suggested alternatives

affect in a positive way	benefit
a number of	many
at this point in time	now
due to the fact that	because
in addition to	also
in the event of	if
prior to	before
male paediatric patient	boy
upper limbs	arms
subsequent to	after

Style: in practice

Clearly there is a huge gap between what the writing 'experts' advocate and what happens in practice (*see* Figure 7.6). The guidelines here are by no means drastic, and applying them should make any piece of writing far more accessible and easy to read. But anyone reading a journal will appreciate that even these basic principles are often ignored.

This can be very confusing for inexperienced writers. From time to time a participant comes to the second day of a training course saying that he or she has written simply, as we suggested, only to find that the professor has changed it all back on the grounds that it was not 'proper scientific writing'.

Luckily there is an easy answer to this problem. For this kind of writing, style is not, and should not be, a way in which we express our personalities. (If you want to do that, try poetry.) It is the way we get information across from one person to another. In this context, style becomes the choice of words and constructions most likely to get the message across to the target audience. This means that the most valuable – indeed the only

---

FIGURE 7.6 Copy-editing in practice

The effect of ~~radiotherapy~~ postoperatively radiotherapy in patients with a positive resection margin will be almost impossible to evaluate ~~in a study since~~ because so few patients are seen in this category. Patients ~~i~~In our group ~~of patients there was no survival advantage for the patients~~ with a positive bronchial resection margin ~~who were~~ treated with radiotherapy survived no longer than those ~~compared to the patients~~ who did not rec~~ei~~ieve it. Local or distal ~~There were no less~~ recurren~~tees, local or distal~~ rates were similar. Others have found this.[1, 2, 3] ~~This observation was also made by others[1, 2, 3]~~.

– criterion of whether a style is 'right' or 'good' is to ask the question: is it appropriate for the target journal?

This in turn means that you should look carefully at the papers the journal publishes, analyse the kind of language and the kind of sentences that are used, and write in that style.

This, of course, is a rational and sensible view. You are about to find that the debate over style becomes a major battleground as your colleagues and your superiors insist that their views are 'better' than yours. What you write will almost certainly be changed, and not always for the best. Try not to waste time getting drawn into what is really quite unimportant detail. Above all, don't take it personally.

✪ CHECKPOINT

Before proceeding to Chapter 8, you should have a manuscript that you feel is ready to be shown to others.

BOOKCHOICE: What is a 'good' style?

Goodman NW, Edwards MB, Langdon-Neuner E (2014) *Medical Writing: a prescription for clarity* (4e). Cambridge University Press, Cambridge.

There are many books on how to write in a good 'scientific' style, and many of them say much the same thing. They wheel out endless lists of what to avoid, such as long sentences, pompous words and the passive voice. The regular publication of these lists, however, seems to have made no difference whatsoever, and daily we see a sharp increase in the volume of papers published in a badly written and often unintelligible style.

But we should not let the trend continue unchallenged. Aspiring writers should read at least one of these books, and I recommend this one. It is now in its fourth edition, having doubled in size over the past 25 years from 180 to 360 pages. It is stuffed full of advice over confused words ('discreet' or 'discrete', 'prescribed' or 'proscribed'); needlessly complicated words ('perform', 'possess', 'predicate') and superfluous phrases ('in respect of', 'it was noted that'). The authors confront the popularity of the passive voice, a persistent cause of friction among co-authors, and come up with a firm view: 'The replacement of passive with active constructions, using personal pronouns where necessary and with effective use of references, makes writing simple and clear.' New in this edition is specific help (written by the third co-author) for the growing number of authors for whom English is not the first language.

The most useful part of the book is the large number of excellent examples that the authors unravel, either in the text or as exercises at the end of the book. For instance:

> *'Despite a plethora of studies on income inequality and health, researchers have been unable to make any firm conclusions as a result of methodological limitations.'*

becomes

'We are still uncertain about the effect of income inequality on health, because of the inadequacy of the methods in many of the numerous studies.'

'Bad writing is contagious if the reader has not received an adequately immunising dose of good,' say the authors. Buy the book and keep it handy. Dip into it when you feel your infection might be returning, or need to boost your efforts to keep your writing clear and healthy. And keep in mind the authors' timely reminder about why you should do it: 'If you forget the conventions of medical writing and just write English, patients will benefit.'

8

Prepare the additional elements

'Breaking the whole into bite-sized chunks has really made me feel that the end goal is achievable.'

The article itself – the text from first word to last – is complete. You have your product; now you have to add to it a number of the additional elements, such as title, abstracts, tables and references. I often used the analogy of marketing a sauce: you have worked out the ingredients, and now you have to add the other parts – such as bottle, cap, label, packaging – that make up the final product.

These 'additionals' can vary from journal to journal, but this should not be a major problem. Look out a copy of your target journal so you can see its preferences. Editors often think they publish their articles in an identical style, but they don't. How do they like their titles? What is the preferred form for figures and tables? Are the abstracts structured? The copy of your target journal should be your guide throughout this coming stage, and the answer to nearly every question about how each element should look is simply: 'A good [title/figure/abstract] is what the editor thinks is a good [title/figure/abstract]'.

If your article is well thought out and with a clear message, adding these elements should not take too much time. For instance, I constantly showed in training courses (often to startled participants) that once the article has been written it takes less than 1 minute to write the title and less than 10 to write the abstract. Some of the other tasks, like checking the references, will take a little longer, but work at it methodically and even these tasks should not be a problem.

The title page

The title page is one of those areas where technology has caused (and is causing) major changes. In the old days (as many as 10 years ago) writers would put a range of vital information, along with the title, on the first page of the manuscript (*see* Figure 8.1). Some still do; others are now led by electronic means to enter all the information that the editors will require. As ever, the answer is to look up the *Instructions to authors*, and do what that tells you. That said, there is a certain amount of information that will be required (*see* Figure 8.2). In addition to the title page, many journals now require authors to complete a conflict of interest notification page (*see* Figure 8.3).

FIGURE 8.1 Title page

Prevalence of post-lunchtime amnesia among doctors in UK hospitals: results of a cross-sectional survey

Andrew W Smith MB BS[1], William AW Smith MD
MRCP[1], Emily S Dupont BSc M Phil[2]

1 Department of Prandiology, New University of
Middleshire, Middleshire, UK
2 Institut Alimentaire, Paris 23, France

Address for correspondence: Dr AW Smith, Room 321,
Department of Prandiology, New University of
Middleshire, Middleshire, UK

This research was undertaken with a grant of £100,000
from the Obecalp Foundation

Running head: Prevalence of PLA in UK hospital doctors

FIGURE 8.2 Requirements on the title page

The title page contains general information about an article and its authors. According to the ICMJE, this information usually includes:

- article title
- author information
- disclaimers
- source(s) of support
- word count
- number of figures and tables

www.icmje.org

FIGURE 8.3 Conflict of interest declaration

These can look silly: *Dr Green once gave a talk to the team developing Obecalp and his wife has 100 shares in the company.* They can also be used to self-advertise: I once saw a declaration of interest that doubled as a free book plug for the authors.

But declarations of conflicts of interest (or what some more gently call 'competing' interests) are extremely important. What matters is not whether you have taken lots of money from the makers of Obecalp (after all, someone has to pay for research) but whether readers are made aware of it – and can make up their own mind accordingly. The current buzzword is 'transparency'. Be guided by the journal – and follow their instructions on conflict of interest to the letter. If in any doubt, ask the editors for advice: they would much rather you did that than find the whole thing blowing up in their faces later on.

The title

This causes an inordinate amount of pain and suffering, probably because it is written in larger letters. Authors and co-authors often become enveloped in the most horrendous rows, even though a paper will almost certainly never be rejected for its title: if the editor doesn't like it, he or she will change it, and often does.

The problem is that there is no consensus on what makes a good title. The ICMJE recommendations state: 'The title provides a distilled description of the complete article and should include information that, along with the abstract, will make electronic retrieval of the article sensitive and specific . . .' This is not particularly helpful, since if you look in a number of journals, you will see a variety of different lengths and styles. Some editors like a string of words: *The prevalence of post-lunchtime amnesia among doctors in UK hospitals*, while others favour brief enigmatic phrases such as *Postlunch dip* or *Two o'clock blues*. Others insist on a colon: *Post-lunchtime amnesia: results of a survey*, and a small minority will favour a verb: *More physicians than surgeons doze off after lunch* (*see* Figure 8.4).

Authors should take a pragmatic approach. From their point of view, the good title is one that the editor approves, without changing. Wait until your article is complete before even thinking about writing it. Research your target journal first, then write the title to fit in with their style. The task should take about 2 minutes. If (or when) your co-authors start suggesting titles that are clearly unsuitable for your target journal, point out to them gently why your version is more acceptable.

	Active verb	Colon	Fewer than 10 words	20 words or more	Mean no. of words in title (s.d.)
FIGURE 8.4 Characteristics of titles in six journals					
N Engl J Med	14	–	11	1	12.1 (±3.8)
*Lancet**	2	7	9	1	13.4 (±4.1)
*BMJ**	3	33	4	10	16.2 (±4.1)
J Pediatr	9	12	12	6	13.6 (±4.9)
Pediatr Res	23	5	7	5	14.3 (±4.3)
*Arch Dis Child**	5	4	26	–	9.8 (±3.5)

*European-based journals.

Source: 50 consecutive articles from 1 June 1997.

Authors

You should normally list the first name, middle initial and last name of each author, with highest academic degree(s) and institutional affiliation. Also list the name of department(s) and institution(s) to which the work should be attributed. That's the easy part.

I warned in Chapter 3 that authorship was a problem area. As the paper approaches publication you will meet more and more pressure from those who see the small part they played as an opportunity to become an author and enhance their CVs (*see* Figure 8.5).

You may also find yourself coming under pressure

FIGURE 8.5 Authorship undermined

Authorship is fast becoming one of the weak points in medical publishing. Editors make it quite clear what they want: a substantial intellectual involvement in the process. University and other administrators have a conflicting demand: that people should clock up as many 'paper points' as they can. This has, not surprisingly, led to a situation where many named authors, quite frankly, are shams. When running courses on writing papers each time I would hear horror stories of people being given gift authorship because their career needed a boost, or because a professor felt he needed to show his power.

This has given medical science a major ethical problem: why should we believe the data when people are blatantly lying (yes, sorry) about their relationship to that data.

That said, junior writers – with no power or influence – have little chance of putting things right. What should they do? The best way forward (as already pointed out in Chapter 3) is to try to agree on authorship before writing the paper – then if people emerge out of the woodwork it does at least look a little obvious and makes it harder for them to press their authorship claims. Failing that, feel free to photocopy this panel and distribute it as required.

---

regarding the order in which the authors are to be listed. The ICMJE recommendations do not really help, stating firmly: 'If agreement cannot be reached about who qualifies for authorship . . . the institution(s) where the work was performed, not the journal editor, should be asked to investigate.' I can only repeat the advice given in Chapter 4 that the best way of avoiding discord and delay is to discuss and agree the order of authors before writing the paper.

Make clear which author is responsible for correspondence about the manuscript and who will be responsible for supplying reprints. Remember that there can be a time lag between acceptance and publication; make sure that your address will still hold true and warn the editor if, for example, you are taking a temporary post overseas. You don't want to delay an already complex publishing process.

Acknowledgements

It is open to question whether it helps readers or advances knowledge to know that Mrs Antrobus helped with the library search. But sometimes debts have to be paid. Whenever possible use a technique of expressing thanks that doesn't detract from this method of communicating science – a box of chocolates, perhaps, or a simple thank-you letter. That said, there are some people whose contributions do need to be recognised (*see* Figure 8.6).

The abstract

An abstract can be a stand-alone item of writing (for presenting at conferences, for instance) but in this case it is a summary. Originally it was the final paragraph of the scientific paper. Then it was moved up to the front of the article where it not only attracts attention to that article, but also satisfies that interest without forcing the reader to plough through the text and tables. It is also used as a 'product' on its own, available in abstract journals and on electronic databases. It follows that the abstract should reflect the article accurately. This sounds like an

---

FIGURE 8.6 The ICMJE recommendations on non author-contributors

'Contributors who meet fewer than all 4 of the above criteria for authorship should not be listed as authors, but they should be acknowledged. Examples of activities that alone (without other contributions) do not qualify a contributor for authorship are acquisition of funding; general supervision of a research group or general administrative support; and writing assistance, technical editing, language editing and proofreading. Those whose contributions do not justify authorship may be acknowledged individually or together as a group . . . and their contributions should be specified . . . Because acknowledgment may imply endorsement by acknowledged individuals of a study's data and conclusions, editors are advised to require that the corresponding author obtain written permission to be acknowledged from all acknowledged individuals.'

www.icmje.org

---

obvious rule, but it is often broken: one well-quoted study found that 18%–68% of abstracts in six major journals had data that were inconsistent with, or absent from, the body of the text.[13]

The ICMJE recommendations give a clear account of what is needed (*see* Figure 8.7). From the writing point of view, consider this as a separate piece of work. Set yourself a brief (*see* Chapter 3). The message will be identical to that of the article, as will the market. The length, however, will be different. Once you have set the brief, collect the information, in this case from your

overnight. Then read it again, compare it with your paper and insert any necessary facts. Adjust the style as required: there is a convention that abstracts are written in the passive voice, and if your target journal favours this style, follow it. This is not the place to campaign for plain English.

References

Strictly speaking, the references are an integral part of the text and not an additional item. You will already have chosen those papers that you wish to cite, and you will probably have gathered a list of some kind, which may look plausible. But put aside some time to check, double-check and tidy up (*see* Figure 8.9).

The responsibility to get it right is yours. The ICMJE recommendations state: '. . . authors should . . . verify references against the original documents'. And herein lies a major problem. A study carried out on four dermatology journals in the USA found that, of all the references cited, about one-third could not be traced, one-third did not say what they were said to have said and only about one-third were accurate.[14] The authors say, with a certain understatement, that this questions the whole business of citing papers.

Check that the papers you cite are doing what they should be doing, which is supporting assertions in the text. If they do not, are you merely engaging in academic name-dropping, which is not what references are for? Even if you do feel it is expedient to cite key papers that have been published previously in your target journal, at

FIGURE 8.9 The ICMJE recommendations on references

'Authors should provide direct references to original research sources whenever possible. References should not be used by authors, editors, or peer reviewers to promote self-interests. Although references to review articles can be an efficient way to guide readers to a body of literature, review articles do not always reflect original work accurately. On the other hand, extensive lists of references to original work on a topic can use excessive space. Fewer references to key original papers often serve as well as more exhaustive lists, particularly since references can now be added to the electronic version of published papers, and since electronic literature searching allows readers to retrieve published literature efficiently.

Do not use conference abstracts as references: they can be cited in the text, in parentheses, but not as page footnotes. References to papers accepted but not yet published should be designated as 'in press' or 'forthcoming'. Information from manuscripts submitted but not accepted should be cited in the text as 'unpublished observations' with written permission from the source.

Avoid citing a 'personal communication' unless it provides essential information not available from a public source, in which case the name of the person and date of communication should be cited in parentheses in the text. For scientific articles, obtain written permission and confirmation of accuracy from the source of a personal communication.

Some but not all journals check the accuracy of all reference citations; thus, citation errors sometimes appear in the published version of articles. To minimize such errors, references should be verified using either an electronic bibliographic source, such as PubMed, or print copies from original sources. Authors are responsible for checking that none of the references cite retracted articles except in the context of referring to the retraction . . .

> References should be numbered consecutively in the order in which they are first mentioned in the text. Identify references in text, tables, and legends by Arabic numerals in parentheses . . .'
>
> www.icmje.org

least it shows a continuing thread. Make sure that they really are relevant.

You should have actually read the papers you cite, and ensured that they say what you say they do. Make sure also that the numbers in the text are the same as the numbers in the list of references, and that there are no discrepancies.

Finally a plea on behalf of professional copy-editors, who say that sorting out references is not only the worst aspect of their job, but also the most time-consuming. Make sure that you follow the style as laid down in the *Instructions to authors*; this doesn't mean simply that the words are roughly in the right order, but that there are not commas where colons should be, and vice versa. Nowadays there is a selection of software that will help you import and collate references, thereby taking out much of the pain that traditionally went with this task. But technology should be an addition to, and not a substitute for, the traditional skill of checking the hard copy yourself.

Tables and figures

You will already have produced your tables and illustrations in rough form. Now is the time to check that these are relevant to and enhance readers' understanding of the text. You must also make sure that they meet the criteria for publication and that numbers in tables match those in the text. The ICMJE recommendations give general guidance (*see* Figure 8.10).

Prepare the figures: the ICMJE recommendations give general guidance (*see* Figure 8.11). Study your target journal's *Instructions to authors* to see if there are any local differences.

Letter to the editor

In the not-so-distant days when manuscripts were sent by parcel post the covering letter was just that – a letter that was placed at the top and gave the first impression. Nowadays, with electronic submission, there are various permutations: some journals will allow you to keep your own letter heading and formatting (by submitting in PDF); others will turn your 'letter' into a formless crush of words; a few may even deny you the chance to submit a letter at all.

As for their usefulness, some editors say they turn to the letter first of all (to see what the authors think is important about their work). Others claim they disregard it. (I take this claim now with a pinch of salt, after one editor told a group I was teaching that editors never read the letter; I was delighted a few months later to see

FIGURE 8.10 The ICMJE recommendations on tables

'Tables capture information concisely and display it efficiently; they also provide information at any desired level of detail and precision. Including data in tables rather than text frequently makes it possible to reduce the length of the text.

Prepare tables according to the specific journal's requirements; to avoid errors it is best if tables can be directly imported into the journal's publication software. Number tables consecutively in the order of their first citation in the text and supply a title for each. Titles in tables should be short but self-explanatory, containing information that allows readers to understand the table's content without having to go back to the text. Be sure that each table is cited in the text.

Give each column a short or an abbreviated heading. Authors should place explanatory matter in footnotes, not in the heading. Explain all nonstandard abbreviations in footnotes, and use symbols to explain information if needed. Symbols may vary from journal to journal (alphabet letter or such symbols as *, †, ‡, §), so check each journal's instructions for authors for required practice. Identify statistical measures of variations, such as standard deviation and standard error of the mean.

If you use data from another published or unpublished source, obtain permission and acknowledge that source fully.

Additional tables containing backup data too extensive to publish in print may be appropriate for publication in the electronic version of the journal, deposited with an archival service, or made available to readers directly by the authors. An appropriate statement should be added to the text to inform readers that this additional information is available and where it is located. Submit such tables for consideration with the paper so that they will be available to the peer reviewers.'

www.icmje.org

FIGURE 8.11 The ICMJE recommendations on illustrations (figures)

'Digital images of manuscript illustrations should be submitted in a suitable format for print publication. Most submission systems have detailed instructions on the quality of images and check them after manuscript upload. For print submissions, figures should be either professionally drawn and photographed, or submitted as photographic quality digital prints.

For X-ray films, scans, and other diagnostic images, as well as pictures of pathology specimens or photomicrographs, send high-resolution photographic image files. Since blots are used as primary evidence in many scientific articles, editors may require deposition of the original photographs of blots on the journal's website.

Although some journals redraw figures, many do not. Letters, numbers, and symbols on figures should therefore be clear and consistent throughout, and large enough to remain legible when the figure is reduced for publication. Figures should be made as self-explanatory as possible, since many will be used directly in slide presentations. Titles and detailed explanations belong in the legends – not on the illustrations themselves.

Photomicrographs should have internal scale markers. Symbols, arrows, or letters used in photomicrographs should contrast with the background. Explain the internal scale and identify the method of staining in photomicrographs.

Figures should be numbered consecutively according to the order in which they have been cited in the text. If a figure has been published previously, acknowledge the original source and submit written permission from the copyright holder to reproduce it. Permission is required irrespective of authorship or publisher except for documents in the public domain.

In the manuscript, legends for illustrations should be on a separate page, with Arabic numerals corresponding to the illustrations. When symbols, arrows, numbers, or letters are used to identify parts of the illustrations, identify and explain each one clearly in the legend.'

www.icmje.org

her reaction when three-quarters of a roomful of editors said they read the letter and found it useful.)

If you do have the opportunity to express yourself in a letter, take a chance that the editor is going to be one who will read it, and make an effort. A good letter will prepare the way for moving the paper forward for further consideration; a bad letter can hasten rejection (*see* Figures 8.12 and 8.13).

A good letter will establish three things:

1. who you are
2. what you are submitting
3. why it should be published.

Publishing an article is to some extent a leap of faith by an editor, so establish your credentials as soon as you can. This is achieved as much by how the letter looks as by the words you use. Use proper headed writing paper. This will establish you as a member of a proper department, and may also give supplementary information, such as department heads, that could strike a positive chord and encourage the editor to trust you.

Lay out the text neatly. Professional communicators have known for some time that the type we use and the

FIGURE 8.12 Letter to the editor: bad example

                                    5 Railway Cuttings
                                       Lower Town
                                       Midshire UK

Dear Sir/Madam,

Please find enclosed one paper on
our recent survey. I am sure you
will agree it is very interesting
indeed.

It is a very important paper, the
first to discover the prevalence
of this condition.

I am an avid reader of your
journal.

Thank you in advance.

AW Smith

FIGURE 8.13 Letter to the editor: better example

Department of Amnesia
University of Wherever
Midtown
England KK8 4LL
From the Professor of Prandiology

Dear Professor Jones,

Prevalence of post-lunchtime amnesia among doctors in UK hospitals: results of a cross-sectional survey

I have pleasure in submitting the above paper for your consideration.

In the last 12 months you have published two papers, one of which came from our team, outlining the devastating effect of individual cases of post-lunchtime amnesia. Our results are the first to show the prevalence of this controversial condition.

I confirm that this article has been read and approved by all the co-authors.

Yours sincerely,

AWS   WAWS   ESDupont

AW Smith   WAW Smith   ES Dupont

way we use it can contribute to whether or not our messages get through. Letters with narrow margins may be seen (unfairly no doubt) to come from people who are unfriendly. Letters with grey type are considered boring. On the other hand those with broad white margins and good black type are considered to be organised and reliable.

Be mindful of the niceties. Address the editor by name – you can easily find this by looking at the publication details. Do not insult the editor by spelling his or her name or title wrong.

Put the title of the paper at the top of your letter. But also explain it in the text, making sure that you use a verb, so that the editor knows what the message is, and not just the subject matter. It will also help your case if you can state tactfully why it should be published. Do not be rude, and say that it's about time the editor published something good. Do not be cute: editors will not be impressed by the fact that you have long enjoyed their journal. Do not offer a bribe. But you can point out that, for instance, the journal has been running a number of articles on this subject and your paper offers an elegant resolution to the debate.

Use the letter also to take care of any legal requirements, such as a statement that the manuscript has been read and approved by all authors. It is also the place to declare any slow-burning bombshells – such as a potential conflict of interest (if not covered elsewhere) or potential redundant publication. If your article has already appeared in, say, another language, and you tell the editor at this stage, there is absolutely no ethical

9

Use internal reviewers

'My boss could do with a course on managing writers effectively.'

'Hit me again . . . and again . . .'

This may be one of the shorter chapters in this book, but it deals with the process that is often the longest and most painful. You will have sweated over your statistics, selected from half a mile of references and agonised over the exact phrasing for a dozen difficult concepts. Now, as you bring your beautiful baby into the world, people are about to tear it limb from limb. And these are the people who are meant to be your friends.

Remain focused on your goal: you want to be a published author. Good advice from other people will be invaluable, essential even. However, much of the advice you get will not necessarily be good, and may even reduce your chances of becoming published. How do you handle this?

One step forward is to divide this process of internal reviewing into two stages: voluntary and compulsory (*see* Figure 9.1). During the voluntary stage you should choose those whose opinions you value and invite their comments in a structured way. You remain free to choose those comments with which you agree. The compulsory stage can come later, and involves showing your manuscript to those whose opinions you are less free to

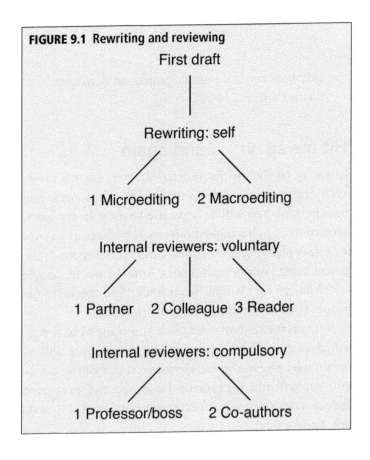

FIGURE 9.1 Rewriting and reviewing

First draft

Rewriting: self

1 Microediting   2 Macroediting

Internal reviewers: voluntary

1 Partner   2 Colleague   3 Reader

Internal reviewers: compulsory

1 Professor/boss   2 Co-authors

discard. These are co-authors and 'bosses'. Your role is to hear what they have to say, accept it when they have something to contribute but negotiate when they are trying to impose changes that, in your view, are going to decrease the chances of becoming published. The second stage, therefore, is more about negotiating skills than writing techniques.

Voluntary reviewing

One of the reasons that this stage can become so unpleasant is the way we approach it. We send off our article to a number of colleagues with a brief note saying 'Any comments?' This is asking for trouble: the only way they can fail in this task is to say nothing. So they make dozens of pencil marks, each of which sears into your soul as a sign of your inadequacy and lack of education.

Choose carefully who you will invite and why. You will probably need four different types of feedback, and therefore you should choose at least one person for each question. When you ask for their help, be specific about what you want them to do, as in the following.

1 To an outsider: Can you spot any stupid mistakes?

We all make basic errors, such as: *The doctors did all they could to elevate the discomfort.* (It should have been *alleviate*.) We therefore need someone with common sense, plus the motivation to catch us out. Partners do this task particularly well. This can be deeply distressing for authors, who have to face the evidence of their

know from your market research is not suited to your target journal. Your only recourse is to show them your evidence, and argue your point with as little emotion as possible.

Then there are professors. What do you do with those who, after you have carefully researched your market and noted that it prefers to use short words and the active voice, carefully change it all back again on the grounds that you are not writing 'scientifically'? In principle, it is better to negotiate than it is to argue or to sulk. Point out what the style of the journal happens to be, and back it up with evidence from that journal. You may not win the argument, but at least you will have tried. (And when you become a professor, you can remember not to fall into the same trap.)

You are unlikely to win every battle. If you are the first author, in theory the decision is yours, though that becomes academic (if you will pardon the pun) if you are a very junior doctor and your critic is a very senior professor. At this stage we are really talking about damage limitation.

---

❷ CHECKPOINT

Before proceeding to Chapter 10 you should have:
- improved your manuscript by taking into account the best comments from a wide range of people
- prevented others from making it unpublishable.

BOOKCHOICE: Taking advice from professionals

Winokur J (ed.) (1999) *Advice to Writers*. Pantheon Books, New York.

If you have got this far you can start calling yourself a writer. So treat yourself to a book giving the views of your new colleagues. This anthology is my long-standing favourite: it will amuse you and help you to improve your writing at the same time. Author Jon Winokur has combed autobiographies, diaries, letters and books to come up with more than 400 bits of advice by writers for writers, arranged in 36 sections from agents and characters to the writer's life and writing tips.

Some of it, such as the sections on agents and dialogue, will not be relevant to the writing of scientific papers, but much of it will be. On general matters, be consoled by John Berryman on reacting to criticism: 'I would recommend the cultivation of extreme indifference to both praise and blame because praise will lead you to vanity, and blame will lead you to self-pity, and both are bad for writers.' Consider James Thurber's 'Don't get it right, get it written' or TS Eliot's 'Whatever you do . . . avoid piles'.

There's good advice on style that will come in useful at this stage. 'A good style must first of all be clear. It must not be mean or above the dignity of the subject. It must be appropriate' (Aristotle). 'When you say something make sure you have said it. The chances of your having said it are only fair' (EB White). Or 'Read over your compositions and when you meet a passage which you think is particularly fine, strike it out' (Samuel Johnson).

There's also some advice on specifics that backs up many of the points made in this book: 'Short words are best and the old words when short are best of all' (Winston Churchill) or 'You should not take hyphens seriously' (Sir Ernest Gowers).

10

Send off the package

'I played the game with the rules you have learned me, and I won . . . As you might notice, my English is not that good but that didn't prevent the paper from being published.'

At last . . .

Finally comes the time when everything is ready and you are about to press the SEND button to convey your masterpiece to your target journal. Resist the temptation. Log onto your target journal's web page (yet again?) and go through the recommendations – including, if you are lucky, a checklist – on how to submit (*see* Figure 10.1). If you have everything . . . press that button.

Coping with rejection

Rare is the author who has not been rejected. When (not if) it happens to you, be as mature as possible. Dry your eyes, leave the rejection letter for a couple of days, then start your post-mortem.

You may wish to blame your rejection on the nature of the reviewing system, but that is a fruitless exercise. You should take responsibility for the failure, though you will find it helpful to ask 'Why did my marketing not succeed this time?' rather than 'Why am I an abject failure?'

One advantage of the reviewing system is that you will usually be told the reasons for rejection. Are the criticisms fair? Can you answer them? Should you consider an appeal? You should certainly not appeal if the letter says something like 'We enjoyed reading your article but we do not feel it is a priority for us at the moment . . .' Reading carefully between the lines will show you that this is a value judgement. The only grounds for appeal would be that you know the editor's job better than he or she. This approach is not likely to win friends and secure publication.

On the other hand, you may feel – and may even be justified in feeling – that the reviewers have misinterpreted what you have said. In this case you have every right to appeal, but do so politely. Do not write and berate the editor for choosing such idiots for reviewers. Do write a considered and polite letter, setting out clearly where you disagree with the reviewers – and what your evidence is. Sometimes your appeal will be upheld.

Another, and more common, alternative is to submit your article elsewhere. Do not simply print out your covering letter again, deleting all references to the editor of *The New England Journal of Medicine* and substituting the name of the editor of the *Transylvanian Annals of Left Handed Surgery*. Re-examine your product carefully. What is your new market and does your message still hold for it? In other words, go back to Chapter 3 and start again. The process should be far quicker this time. Be encouraged by the fact that most rejected papers eventually get published.

Throughout your dealings with editors and reviewers, do as you would be done by. It's a bit like the doctor–patient relationship, though this time you are the patient. There are striking similarities between a nightmare patient and a nightmare writer: refusal to admit error, persistency, reluctance to take advice.

Of course, there comes a time in every task when we have to admit that it won't succeed. But when do you know when to stop submitting? The answer is relatively straightforward. When you start getting the same kind of objections from the reviewers and you are unable to meet them, then you should call it a day. And channel your energies into another paper.

Coping with acceptance

So much for the gloom. There will almost certainly come a time when you reach the promised land and find that an article you have written has been accepted. This is likely to be a qualified acceptance, if only because editors and reviewers feel that they are failing in their job if they don't criticise. But there will be a clear implication – even a firm promise – that they will publish your paper provided you make the recommended changes. Make sure that you do these changes as quickly as possible. I often meet people who have interpreted a qualified acceptance as a rejection, thereby missing out on the chance of publication.

You can start to rejoice as your article moves towards the process of publication. But even at this stage there are one or two pitfalls lying ahead.

Be careful of prior publication. Some journals will not publish anything that has been published elsewhere. The nightmare scenario is that your paper is being prepared for publication, and at the same time you are giving a presentation to a conference. There is present an astute reporter from a lay paper, who recognises the important implications of what you have done – and, as their job requires them to do, writes it up accordingly. In theory, your paper, though accepted, could now be rejected. The best way of dealing with this is to liaise in advance with the editor. Let him or her know what is happening, and there should be no problems.

You should soon receive a proof of your article. Do not be surprised if it differs from your version. That is because all publications have someone whose job it is to copy-edit all articles. They will carry through a number of checks. They will – if they have time, which most of them increasingly say they have not – carry out some stylistic changes in order to make your article more suitable for their target audience.

Trust their judgement: they will normally have considerable experience at their job, plus detailed knowledge of the demands of their readership. Do not be over-proprietorial with what you have written and under no circumstances should you reinstate your version word for word.

On the other hand, do not just tick the proof without reading it. Check it carefully for accuracy. Look for the obvious spelling mistakes. Check the numbers. Look at dosages and check names and titles. Make sure you meet any deadlines.

After publication

Now is the time to forget the pain. You are about to become a Published Author. Enjoy the experience. You will have earned it.

Take a short rest, then work out whether you want to get back to healing the sick – or start all over again.

> If you have got this far, you should have become a published author. Make sure you celebrate.

biological and medical sciences. Cambridge University Press, Cambridge.

12. Smith R (1996) 'Since this paper was written the death of one of the authors has occurred'. *Short Words*, TAA Training, Leatherhead.

13. Pitkin RM, Branagen MA and Burmeister LF (1999) Accuracy of data in abstracts of published research articles. *JAMA*. **281**: 1110–11.

14. George PM and Robbins K (1994) Reference accuracy in the dermatologic literature. *J Am Acad Dermatol*. **31**: 61–4.

15. Whimster WF (1997) *Biomedical Research: how to plan, publish and present it*. Springer, London.

Some useful
websites

www.equator-network.org: Checklists and guidelines for reporting different kinds of studies.

http://scholarlyoa.com/publishers: List of 'potential, possible, or probable predatory' open access publishers.

www.plainenglish.co.uk: This site, provided by pioneers of straightforward English, is great fun, and includes a facility for finding alternatives to jargon words.

www.biosemantics.org/jane/: JANE stands for journal/author name estimator, and if you feed in your proposed title (or key words) this resource aims to 'find the best matching journals, authors or articles'.

www.icmje.org/recommendations: The full text of the principles as set down by leading medical journal editors. It changes from time to time so is worth keeping an eye on.

http://publicationethics.org/files/Code_of_conduct_for_journal_editors.pdf: These are the principles which editors are urged to uphold.

www.exeter.ac.uk/research/openaccess/: Good information on open access, the growing movement from funders and others that research should be freely available.

www.sherpa.ac.uk/romeo: Information on how journals are complying with open access requests.

http://retractionwatch.com: A salutary site, giving (sometimes hilarious) details of papers that have gone wrong, by accident or design.

www.timalbert.co.uk: Information about the author, the courses he devised, some additional advice and a list of trainers who are accredited to run the Writing a Scientific Paper – and Getting it Published course.

Index

Entries in *italics* denote figures.

fear of, 63–4
finding time for, 19, 65–6
fleshing out, 41–2
goals for, 17, *18*
lifestyle of, 15–16
objectives for, 19–20
preparatory stages of, 21–4
principles of effective, 4–5

process of, 1–3
schedule for, 34, *35*
in short bursts, 67
structure of, 51
see also scientific writing
writing team, *36*

'yellow marker' test, 74, 77

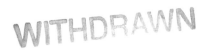